RC
280
.B8
G72
1988

Greenberg, Mimi.

Invisible scars

$17.95

DATE			

© THE BAKER & TAYLOR CO.

INVISIBLE
SCARS

A Guide to

Coping with the

Emotional Impact

of Breast Cancer

INVISIBLE SCARS

A Guide to
Coping with the
Emotional Impact
of Breast Cancer

MIMI GREENBERG, Ph.D.

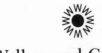

Walker and Company
New York

First published in the United States of America in 1988 by the Walker Publishing Company, Inc.

Published simultaneously in Canada by Thomas Allen & Son Canada, Limited, Markham, Ontario.

Library of Congress Cataloging-in-Publication Data

Greenberg, Mimi
  Invisible scars.

  Bibliography: p.
  Includes index.
  1. Breast—Cancer—Psychological aspects. 2. Adjust-
ment (Psychology) 3. Women—Psychology. I. Title.
RC280.B8G72 1988   616.99′499′0019   88-19
ISBN 0-8027-1020-4

Printed in the United States of America

10 9 8 7 6 5 4 3 2 1

Contents

Dedication

*I*n loving memory of my father, Kenneth, who encouraged me to write this book but did not live long enough to see it completed. Popsie, your spirit is always with me.

Author's Note

*F*or the sake of literary uniformity, the physician is referred to as *he*. I am fully aware that women are represented in every medical specialty and that many of us are being treated by highly qualified general surgeons, reconstructive surgeons, oncologists, and radiotherapists who are women.

Foreword

Invisible Scars is a book that desperately needed to be written. Until now, there was no practical guide for understanding and coping with the emotional impact of breast cancer.

Invisible Scars fills that void. It is a wonderful, uplifting book for the woman who has just discovered she has breast cancer as well as for the woman who has completed all of her treatment and is now concerned with recovery. Each chapter facilitates understanding and helps resolve the emotional turbulence that accompanies diagnosis, treatment, and recovery.

Dr. Greenberg takes you by the hand, walks you through the emotional pitfalls, and teaches you how to handle each of them. Using examples from patients, she gives you the psychological tools to use if you want to reduce the turmoil and assume more control over your life. She even goes into the types, pros and cons, and monetary costs of psychological counseling. The vicissitudes of maintaining or getting health insurance coverage are weighed as well.

Only a woman who has been treated for this disease and who has successfully dealt with her own emotions could express herself so empathically. Mimi is a licensed psychologist who is able to reflect on her feelings and experiences as a breast cancer patient in a way that helps others accept and deal effectively with their own fears.

This book is warm with humor and understanding. The feelings, decisions, and needs of the patient become real. It takes you through emotional basics. It teaches you when to speak up, to whom, how, where, and when; at the end of each chapter there is an easy summary to make sure you understood the main points.

Mimi's writing style is friendly, caring, and direct . . . the way you would like your mother, sister or best friend to talk to you. She tells you about situations and feelings everyone who has breast cancer undergoes and how to resolve them. Some are universal, unavoidable, and must be faced, and others can be avoided for they are self- or society-inflicted.

Her advice is excellent, for it lets you know that you are not alone. She makes sensible suggestions as to how to cope with yourself, your partner, doctors, friends, coworkers, and even your boss. She tells it straight . . . and you will feel better for having read those passages.

This book will be given as immediate required reading to all of my patients who receive a diagnosis of breast cancer.

Penny Wise Budoff, M.D.
Author—*No More Hot Flashes and Other Good News*

Acknowledgments

*T*here are a number of thank-yous I would like to make. The first is to Edward H. Phillips, M.D., F.A.C.S., oncological surgeon, Cedars-Sinai Medical Center, Los Angeles, California, for his insight into the emotional needs of women with breast cancer and his commitment to make psychological support available to all of his patients, regardless of their financial means.

I want to thank Leslie Botnick, M.D., Director of Radiation Oncology, St. Joseph's Medical Center, Burbank, California, for being a "mensch extraordinaire" and for always making time to talk, teach, and go out of his way to help.

Melvin J. Silverstein, M.D., Medical Director of the Breast Center in Van Nuys, California. He and the Breast Center Staff, which includes James R. Waisman, M.D.; Parvis Gamagami, M.D.; Bernard S. Lewinsky, M.D.; Aaron G. Fingerhut, M.D.; Neal Handel, M.D.; Eugene D. Gierson, M.D.; Robert J. Rosser, M.D.; William J. Colburn, M.D.; Patricia S. Gordon, M.D.; Ellen L. Waisman, B.S.; and Barbara J. Brighton, M.A., have provided me with a firm background and understanding of the medical issues from which springs a plethora of psychological problems.

Penny Wise Budoff, M.D., gynecologist, researcher, author, and founder of the Penny Wise Budoff, M.D. Women's Medical Center in Bethpage, New York, for writing the book *No More Hot Flashes, And Other Good News.* Her chapter on breast cancer was my greatest source of comfort and reassurance that the treatment choice I was about to make was the right one for me.

Michael Van Scoy-Mosher, M.D., medical oncology, Cedars-Sinai Medical Center, Los Angeles, California, for making me feel welcome at Cedars' breast tumor board, and for being a fine sounding board whenever I have needed one.

Wendy Schain, Ed.D., Medical Care Consultant, National Institute of Health, Bethesda, Maryland, and Rose Kushner, author, and Executive Director of the Breast Cancer Advisory Center, Kensington, Maryland, whom I first knew as role models and later as friends, gave generously of their time and made many valuable suggestions. Thanks to Nancy Bruning, whom I first approached to coauthor this book and who, instead, wisely offered me the encouragement, friendship, and support to make this a solo effort.

I am grateful to Irwin Grossman, M.D., Medical Director of Spalding Radiology Center, Beverly Hills, California; Saar Porrath, M.D., Medical Director of The Woman's Breast Center, Santa Monica, California; David D. Hopp, M.D., plastic and reconstructive surgery, Cedars-Sinai Medical Center, Los Angeles, California; Janet Salomonson, M.D., plastic and reconstructive surgery, Santa Monica, California; Becky J. Miller, M.D., medical oncology, Los Angeles, California; David Wellisch, Ph.D., Associate Professor of Medical Psychology, UCLA Neuropsychiatric Hospital, Los Angeles, California; and Cathy Coleman, R.N., Administrative Director, Long Beach Memorial Breast Evaluation Center, Long Beach, California.

Numerous medical oncologists on the staff at Cedars-Sinai Medical Center contributed to the background, preparation, and completion of this book. They include: Barry E. Rosenbloom, M.D.; Robert J. Taub, M.D.; R. Clifford Ossorio, M.D.; Melvin Avedon, M.D.; and Laurence J. Heifetz, M.D.

Many good friends served as readers and gave emotional support. They include: Bernice Kotkin, Ph.D.; Alice Koenigsberg; Linda Turer-Orenstein; Corky McClellan; Candy Johnson; Sally Taub; Beth Grossman-Aubrey; Sandy Meyer; Bob Carson; Wendy Tucker; Tom Lehn; Lee Colomby; and Wendy Brandchaft.

I would like to express my appreciation for the help and support from my editor, Richard Winslow, as well as my agent, Susan Ann Protter.

And especially to all of my patients, past and present, I'm grateful.

Finally, I will always be indebted to William Grace, M.D., Chief of Medical Oncology, St. Vincent's Hospital and Medical Center of New York, and Steven I. Neibart, M.D., for their kindness and humanity toward my father and me during his final weeks.

Introduction

I never thought I would write a book on breast cancer. Then again, I never thought I would *have* breast cancer. And if it ever did fleetingly cross my mind, I never considered how I would think, feel, and react—or what I might do to make the diagnosis, treatment, and recovery less of an emotional ordeal. In 1983 I found out, firsthand.

Shocked, confused, crying, pounding pillows one minute, composed and serene the next, the once confident and self-assured psychologist who was used to solving everyone else's problems crumbled into a fragile, frightened creature who felt totally alone and alienated from the world. That is how I began my odyssey into the world of breast cancer.

My experience as a patient was filled with tension and emotional turmoil. Much of it was unnecessary. The visible surgical scars were nothing compared to the invisible emotional scars. My background as a psychotherapist in private practice since 1975 made me aware that much of this trauma was avoidable, and could have been prevented or at least minimized if I had understood the psychological issues before they caught me on my blind side. Also, it would have helped if I had been in psychotherapy with someone who had successfully recovered from breast cancer.

I needed support, guidance, and a role model. I muddled through, as most of us do, with the help of family and friends—whose well-meaning intentions upset me as often as they comforted me.

I promised myself that when I fully recovered (physically and emotionally), I would integrate my personal experience with my professional skills and become the psychotherapist I had searched for and never found. This was easier said than done.

Initially, the medical community was skeptical of my skills and intentions. Undaunted, I began reading breast cancer literature and attending breast tumor board meetings at various hospitals. (At breast tumor boards breast cancer cases, such as yours and mine, are presented to the medical community for discussion.) I listened carefully to what was being said and why. Sometimes, I put in my two cents about the psychological impact of breast cancer, just as a reminder that I was still around and very much interested and dedicated to the subject matter. Some doctors may have felt like I was a pesky fly at a picnic. Because they couldn't get rid of me, they ignored me. Occasionally someone acknowledged my presence saying there were no psychological issues that couldn't be handled by the physician. Some said there were no psychological issues period! I was appalled . . . personally and professionally.

Without the assistance of the medical community, how would patients know that professional psychological help was available from someone who lived through it?

One year later I figured it out. The media! With their help, I decided to launch a consumer awareness campaign on "The Emotional Impact of Breast Cancer" consisting of TV, radio, newspaper, and magazine interviews. It worked! Breast cancer patients began responding enthusiastically. They came in for therapy and then went back to their doctors, saying they were learning how to cope with the emotional impact of breast cancer by talking to a psychologist who had been there too. The patients were educating their physicians, and the physicians were listening to what they had to say!

That is how I began to acquire an air of legitimacy in the medical community. Today, most of my patients are referred by their doctors, but I still welcome calls from women who are self-referred.

As my work with patients progresses, I see similar themes and issues emerging from woman to woman. I also notice that I am invariably asked if there is a book they can read that focuses specifically on the psychological aspects of breast cancer. I finally grew weary of shaking my head no and decided to write one myself.

This is a book that would have been a great help and comfort to me and to my patients when each of us began grappling with the emotional impact of breast cancer.

This book is intended as a self-help tool to be used primarily by you throughout your diagnosis, treatment, and recovery. Your family, friends, and health-care workers may find it helpful too, in better understanding you and your feelings.

It would be impossible to anticipate every potential psychological problem that you may encounter as a breast cancer patient. But don't worry. The same psychological principles and ideas discussed in these chapters can be applied to other problems and issues you may face. In fact, if you are unable to participate in individual psychotherapy or can't find a support group in your town, you may want to use this book as your basic source of emotional support.

An Overview

of the

Psychological

Problems

*T*here are two types of psychological problems we experience as breast cancer patients:

UNAVOIDABLE: Those that come with the turf, so to speak, in that they are universal and innate to the breast cancer experience. In this category are the fears of dying; disfigurement; rejection by husband/lover, family, friends, or business associates; and loss of control over your life. If the bad news is that these fears are unavoidable, the good news is they are controllable.

AVOIDABLE: The second category of problems does not come with the turf and is therefore created unnecessarily (but most of us never realize it). I am referring to the emotional upsets and traumas inadvertently caused by the words and actions of the people around us—specifically, our doctors, their staffs, and, not infrequently, our families, friends, co-workers, and sometimes, ourselves.

How does an avoidable problem occur? Essentially, someone says or does something that upsets us. Instead of telling the person, which would clear up the misunderstanding before it mushrooms into a problem, we withdraw, deny, or minimize our feelings. By our silence, we wind up feeling hurt, angry, depressed, and misunderstood. In other words, the way we respond determines whether we will prevent or experience an avoidable problem.

When we keep upsetting feelings to ourselves, we experience avoidable problems. When we acknowledge and express these feelings, we prevent them.

There is one catch, however: First, we must be in touch with *what we are feeling.* One of the goals of this book is to make us more aware of our feelings so that we can speak up in an appropriate way, in order to solve or, better yet, avoid these problems.

Avoidable problems occur when:

- Someone who intends to be helpful during the course of our diagnosis, treatment, or recovery does or says something that upsets us.

- We are afraid to tell the person how we feel and, instead, emotionally withdraw.

- The person is oblivious to his/her words or actions and can't figure out why we are now acting aloof.

- This makes us feel even more alienated, alone, and overwhelmed. We are convinced that if we didn't have breast cancer, none of these problems would have occurred.

Let's look at an example of an avoidable problem inadvertently caused by a doctor:

ALICE—Alice was lying in the hospital bed postreconstructive surgery. She was eagerly waiting for her plastic surgeon to remove the bandages. The surgeon entered, removed the dressing, and proudly stated that he had created a work of art. Satisfied with the results, he replaced the dressing and left. Alice was stunned. He hadn't asked how *she* felt about her new breast. His seeming lack of interest in her feelings caused her to emotionally withdraw from the doctor and cry silently to herself. For the remainder of her hospital stay she was depressed.

Alice's depression and withdrawal from her doctor were avoidable. In other words, it could have been prevented if a) the doctor had been more aware and sensitive to Alice's feelings, or b) Alice had been more open with the doctor and told him how his behavior affected her.

Did it occur to Alice to tell the doctor how she felt? Of course it did. Why didn't she speak up? She was afraid the doctor would become angry or impatient and this would ultimately lead to receiving inferior medical treatment from him. Does this sound far-fetched? It isn't. I hear it all the time from patients. In fact, this is the most frequent reason given to me by breast cancer patients as to why they don't tell their doctors when they are unhappy with what the doctors have said or done.

Sometimes a member of the doctor's staff will say or do something upsetting:

BRENDA—On the second day of her radiation treatment, Brenda noticed one of the male technicians staring at her breast. At first she thought it was her imagination, but when this continued for several days, she became convinced that it was not a fantasy. She felt intimidated and scared by the technician and contemplated dropping out of radiation treatment or seeking it elsewhere.

Brenda's feelings of intimidation by the technician and her plan to interrupt her treatment were avoidable. In other words, this problem could have been prevented if a) the technician had been more aware of her discomfort, or b) Brenda had told him how she felt.

Did she say anything? No. Why? Because she was afraid it would only make matters worse. She thought the technician would deny staring at her breast and then she would appear foolish and dishonest in front of her doctor.

Even well-meaning family members can inadvertently create unnecessary problems and tension:

CARLA—Carla's parents had been divorced for many years when she found out about the breast cancer diagnosis. The day Carla told them, each reacted by accusing the other of having a history of breast cancer on that side of the family. Carla felt angry because no one was listening to her. She wasn't looking for a culprit to blame. She was looking for emotional support.

Did she tell them how she felt? No. Why? She was afraid they would stop loving her. Instead, she clammed up whenever either parent would phone or visit.

Carla's anger at her parents and the decision to remain silent in order to maintain their love were avoidable if a) Carla's parents had been more empathic to her situation, or b) Carla had been willing to let her parents know how their behavior had hurt her.

Friends and co-workers can unintentionally add to our turmoil and not realize it:

DENISE—Denise confided in her close friend Kim that she was in chemotherapy treatment. In an effort to rally support for Denise, Kim passed on the information to others.

It got back to Denise and she was horrified. She felt betrayed by a friend who had gossiped behind her back.

Did Denise tell Kim how she felt? No. Why? She was afraid of losing the friendship. Instead, she swallowed the feelings and avoided Kim.

Denise's feeling of betrayal and her decision to stay away from her friend were avoidable. In other words, this problem could have been prevented if a) Kim had been more thoughtful of Denise's feelings or b) Denise had been willing to tell her friend how she felt about her actions.

When I first met these four women, each felt she had no control over her problem, she was at the mercy of people who were insensitive to her feelings, and there was no constructive way to avoid or repair the situation. Actually the opposite was true.

Avoidable problems can be prevented when:

> • The other person is especially sensitive and empathic to our feelings during diagnosis, treatment, and recovery. Or . . .

> • We are willing to tell the other person what he/she said or did that was upsetting.

Avoidable problems can be solved or repaired when:

> • We realize there is always at least one constructive solution to any situation and sometimes there are several.

- We accept that most people want to respond sensitively to us, but may not be aware of our feelings.

- We approach the problem logically. We know darn well what caused the problem, how we feel about it, and what it would take to make it better. This automatically gives us the control (if we are willing to accept it).

It's up to us to address the problem and thereby resolve it.

Usually it is harder to avoid the problem than to repair it. Why? Because we have no control over what the people around us say and do. But all is not lost. We can teach them to become more aware, and ultimately this helps us. Benevolent education is a critical factor in preventing avoidable problems. This book is intended to help accomplish that task. If there are sections that are particularly meaningful to you, make note of them and ask the significant people in your life to read these passages, so that you can discuss the material together. When you do this, you will find a new level of understanding and intimacy developing between you. And the number of avoidable problems will be fewer and farther between.

There is no reason to maintain and support our own unhappiness and other people's ignorance, when we have the power to change the situation. It is clear that many problems could have been avoided if the individuals had only known better. But how will anyone ever know better, unless we begin to tell them?

What is the difference between avoiding and repairing a problem? Timing. *Avoiding* is when we address the problem immediately (or as soon as it is reasonably possible) without stewing over it. *Repairing* is when we thrash the problem around for a while (possibly creating new conflicts in addition to the original one) before we solve the matter.

Avoiding or repairing problems is based on three principles:

COURAGE: To make our own needs and feelings our top priority during the course of diagnosis, treatment, and recovery.

CONVICTION: To recognize that if we don't attend to our own needs and feelings, our emotional recovery from breast cancer will be unnecessarily difficult and lengthy.

CANDOR: To be forthright, first, with ourselves in identifying our needs and feelings. Second, with others in communicating these needs and feelings honestly and directly.

The main point is to recognize when someone or something is bothering you and then give yourself permission to say so. But *when* and *how* is the question. Do you speak up immediately or do you mull it over first? This is "The Sooner or Later Syndrome." Ideally, sooner is better than later. But there are always exceptions:

• If you are not used to speaking up for yourself (most of us aren't), you may feel fumbling and awkward. If you prefer to clarify your thoughts before communicating them, that's perfectly reasonable. One word of caution: since this is a new game plan for you, it's natural to feel uncomfortable the first few times up at bat (no matter how much you practice what you want to say). So don't wait too long or you may lose your courage.

• If you have a hot temper, cool down first. Tantrums and abusive language rarely, if ever, produce desired results. Your complaints will be clearer and more effective if you are calm. And they are also more likely to be taken seriously rather than written off as those of "another hysterical female."

• If there are other people present, wait for them to leave. There is no need to involve others in a one-to-one discussion. Your feelings are legitimate. You don't need an audience or a Greek chorus to back you up.

I advocate acting sooner (avoiding) instead of later (re-pairing) because I don't believe in suffering. Especially unnecessarily. There is already too much of that associated with breast cancer. In addition, acting sooner is the quick-est way to regain the sense of control you thought you had lost (or never felt you had in the first place).

The women in our four examples suffered needlessly because they felt helpless in their relationships and hope-less about solving their situations without causing even more damage. That is why they came for psychotherapy. During the course of treatment, each woman was able to successfully repair the problem without harming herself or others. And in so doing, she created a healthy balance in the very relationship she feared would be made worse. You can learn from their experiences.

Let's see how each woman dealt with the issues in a more constructive manner and was able to repair the problem or relationship that was stressful to her.

Repairing the Problem with the Doctor

ALICE didn't want her doctor to think she was criticizing him. But she realized she could never feel right about him unless she discussed what was upsetting her. She decided it would be a lot easier to tell him what was wrong if she also included what was right. This was a diplomatic ap-proach that was also genuine and heartfelt.

The doctor realized his error without becoming defensive and was sincerely appreciative for the honest feedback. The relationship became more comfortable for Alice because she now knew that her doctor was approachable and really cared about her feelings. Not surprisingly, her depression lifted.

Repairing the Problem with the Doctor's Staff

BRENDA felt she couldn't prove the technician was staring at her, so it was useless to complain. She soon came to realize that the real issue wasn't whether he was staring at her, but rather that she felt uncomfortable around him. She accepted that it was her right and privilege to request that this particular technician not be involved in her treatment.

Once Brenda realized that she wasn't at the mercy of the technician and she did have control over the situation—if she was willing to be assertive—she felt better about herself and was able to approach the doctor with her request and without feeling foolish. The doctor agreed to the request, Brenda was relieved that she hadn't interrupted her treatment, and there was no further incident with the technician.

Was there any other constructive solution? Yes. Another option was to talk directly to the technician (e.g., "Sometimes I think you are staring at me and I feel uncomfortable"). In all likelihood, the problem would have stopped right then and there (regardless of whether it was real or imagined), and she would not have needed to take it further.

Is one solution better than the other? Not really. Some of us like to go right to the top when we have a problem. Others prefer to resolve it on a more personal level, going to the top only as a last resort.

Since Brenda was on the verge of quitting treatment, she made a wise choice in taking it directly to her doctor. If the situation had not already reached crisis proportions,

I would have encouraged her to consider speaking with the technician first.

Repairing the Problem with Family Members

CARLA realized that much of her childhood and adult life was spent in the role of arbitrator for her parents' domestic squabbles. When she needed their help, they were always physically present but emotionally absent. She was angry with them for being self-centered and unable to hear how scared and alone she felt.

Despite her trepidation, she mustered up the courage to say that she needed their emotional support but not their personal grievances against each other. The essence of her message was "I don't have the energy to cope with *your* battles and *my* breast cancer at the same time."

Carla's parents were jarred into reality. As a result, they changed their behavior for the remainder of her treatment and recovery. This made it possible for Carla to receive and her parents to give the nurturing and love she needed.

Repairing the Problem with Friends and Co-Workers

DENISE didn't want to further strain the friendship by questioning why her friend had gossiped to others about her chemotherapy. Yet she knew she would never again trust Kim unless she found out her true motives. Was Kim genuinely concerned with her welfare or simply interested in passing on a juicy tidbit?

Denise realized she couldn't avoid her friend forever and so she cautiously posed the question. It turned out that Kim was motivated by anxiety—that if this could happen to Denise, it could happen to her too. She was looking for emotional support and comfort for both of them. Although her judgment left much to be desired, Kim truly meant no malice and felt miserable that she had hurt her friend.

Denise knew Kim was being honest with her. Although she still wished that her friend had been less panicky and more practical, she understood how terrified Kim was at the threat of breast cancer. She accepted the apology and the friendship was restored.

Denise also came to grips with another reality: Having breast cancer is big news to the people who know you, whether you're a Hollywood movie star or a housewife from Hackensack. It's not terribly realistic to think you will tell just a few close friends and no one else will find out. I'm certainly not advocating that friends should breach our confidences. I'm just making an observation about human nature and breast cancer, based on many patients' experiences, including my own.

It is impossible to anticipate every avoidable problem that might be encountered during breast cancer *diagnosis, treatment,* and *recovery.* However, there are some that occur with greater frequency than others.

Diagnosis

The One-Step Procedure

This is a process in which you may be asked to sign a form agreeing to the surgical removal of your breast if a malignancy is found during the biopsy procedure. The reason it is called "one-step" is that both the biopsy and mastectomy are performed in one procedure or "step." You do not know at the time the anesthesia is administered if you have breast cancer. The only way to find out is after you wake up and put your hand to your chest. If your breast is missing, you know you had cancer. There is no period of emotional adjustment between diagnosis and surgery. And, clearly, there is no opportunity to get a second opinion prior to treatment.

Most doctors recognize the emotionally destructive potential of the one-step procedure and don't suggest it to their patients. But every once in a while I meet a woman who was offered and accepted a one-step procedure because she was told that "it saves time and money." Need I tell you that these women find their emotional recovery from breast cancer more difficult and complicated? Why? As most of us know, adjusting to the diagnosis is difficult enough without simultaneously having to cope with the loss of a breast (or two). And there is always a remote possibility that an error was made in either the diagnosis or treatment recommended. Therefore, getting a second opinion is both medically and psychologically sound.

How do you avoid becoming a psychological casualty of the one-step procedure? First, you say *"No"* if it is offered to you. Second, you go to another doctor—one who is more sensitive and aware of women in general, and of you in particular.

Second Opinions

The purpose of a second opinion is to protect us from misdiagnosis, as well as from unnecessary or incorrect treatment. Theoretically, it should provide medical and psychological reassurance. Most of the time it does. But occasionally it fails. For example:

Split Recommendations

Sometimes the doctors don't agree on the treatment of choice for your particular type, stage, and size of breast cancer. And, in fact, they may vehemently disagree and tell you things about breast cancer and each other that you wish you had never heard and are also irrelevant:

> EVELYN was told by doctor #1 that unless she opted for a mastectomy she could expect to die within ten years. Doctor #2 told her she was an excellent candidate for breast-saving procedures (lumpectomy and radiation). Each physician expressed disdain for the other's recommendation. Whom was she supposed to believe? By the time she got into psychotherapy, she was confused, frightened, and too suspicious to trust anyone's opinion.

How can you prevent this from happening to you? Get opinions and recommendations from breast cancer specialists. Their knowledge is more apt to be state-of-the-art than that of someone who occasionally treats breasts (such as your internist or gynecologist).

When I was diagnosed by a breast cancer specialist, another doctor friend disagreed with the recommendation and urged me to elect more extensive treatment. Although well meaning, he knew little about current methods. As a result, it created a great deal of anxiety and havoc in my life. Finally, I talked with a second breast cancer specialist who reassured me that the original recommendation was sound. This was one of the first (but hardly the last) of my experiences with avoidable problems!

How can we reduce the anxiety that accompanies a "split recommendation"?

1. Consider the source. Specifically, avoid doctors who have a smattering of breast cancer knowledge that may be twenty to thirty years behind the time. Instead, go to the specialists.

2. Trust your own gut instinct—especially if the experts can't agree on a plan. It beats flipping a coin to decide which one is right.

3. Go for a third opinion. However, if you do this, please remember that you are not conducting a Gallup poll. Resist the temptation to gather so many opinions that you wind up back where you started—confused and indecisive.

Treatment

Physical Side Effects

Regardless of the treatment we choose, there are short- and long-term physical side effects that are important to know about *before we start treatment.* Why? Physical side effects can produce emotional side effects. When we know what they are and what to expect, they become less awesome and we feel more in control.

FRANCINE, like most women receiving radiation treatment, was experiencing fatigue. If someone had told her that fatigue is one of the side effects of radiation treatment, she would have prepared for it (by rearranging her sleep schedule to include an extra hour, or keeping her work schedule free of extra projects, as well as her social calendar free of excessive commitments). But she was not given this information, and so when she became unusually tired, she got scared and was certain the treatment wasn't working and that the cancer had returned.

In Francine's case, the avoidable problem was caused by something that *wasn't* said or done. Important information wasn't given to her.

What can we do to avoid/reduce the emotional complications that accompany the physical side effects?

1. Don't wait for the doctor or staff to give you information on treatment side effects. Ask for it *before* you make treatment choices. It will provide important and useful input that will help you to reach an informed decision.

2. Request that the information be in written form so that you can easily refer to it. If it isn't, tell your doctor you would like a pamphlet or fact sheet describing the various treatments you are considering and their side effects.

3. If you don't understand something you've read, ask the doctor for clarification.

Appointments

Appointments for treatment need to be scheduled at mutually convenient times. If the appointment time isn't good for you, don't set it, because:

1. If you keep the appointment, you are apt to feel angry, begrudging, or, worse, like a martyr.

2. If you break the appointment (especially without a good reason) you are apt to feel guilty, and you may also compromise the results if your treatment is based on specific timed intervals (as in chemotherapy or radiation). It may take a little more time and effort to find a workable appointment schedule, but it's worth it. After all, it's your treatment, your life, and your right to make it reasonably convenient for yourself.

A Few Hints on Scheduling Appointments That Will Help You Eliminate Avoidable Problems:

1. Before you commit to treatment with a specific doctor, find out the schedule availability so that:

• You can rework your schedule to accommodate the appointment times available.

• The staff can reschedule existing appointments to accommodate your schedule.

• If nothing can be worked out, you will still have ample time to go elsewhere without compromising your health.

2. Don't schedule appointments at times that are potentially difficult (such as close to when you drop your kids off at school or have a weekly staff meeting at the office). You will feel unnecessarily pressured and resentful of everyone and everything.

Recovery

Timetables

Some of us feel the need to live up to other people's expectations of how long it should take to recover from breast cancer. When we use someone else's timetable as our own, we wind up creating emotional chaos.

Although the doctor advised GERRI to wait six weeks before returning to work, she didn't listen. Three weeks after her mastectomy, she was back at her desk because her boss said the work was piling up and what difference would it make whether she sat at home or in the office. Gerri found out that it made a big difference. Within a few days, she was exhausted, had pulled her back and shoulder muscles, and was in such severe physical pain that she couldn't return to work for eight weeks. Additionally, she now had to go to physical therapy for her injured back and shoulder. When I first met her she was depressed over the added delay in returning to work, as well as angry with herself for following her boss's timetable instead of her own.

The flip side of the same problem is that well-meaning family members or friends may unwittingly encourage us to malinger, to take a much longer time to recover than we really need. Before we know it, we become self-imposed invalids who feel helpless and hopeless.

How can we avoid buying into someone else's timetable for our recovery?

1. Listen to the doctor and follow instructions. Doctors really do know the recovery timetable better than your boss, family, or friends.

2. Don't assume that your recovery rate will be identical to that of other breast cancer patients you know, or that other breast cancer patients know more than the doctor about your speed of recovery.

3. Again, trust your instincts. If you're not sure whether you're ready to return to work, you're probably not. But if you insist, try a half-day and see how you fare. You can always build up your hours *slowly*.

I have heard patients say they are positive their employers will not permit gradual reentries back to work. When I encourage them to ask anyway, they usually discover their employers are willing to arrange this without fuss or fanfare.

Psychologically, a gradual reentry is important because it allows you to experience success and a sense of control, rather than prematurely returning to work full time and then experiencing grand failure and depression.

Resuming Sexual Activity

Some of us put too much emphasis on which partner makes the first move to resume sexual activity. We attribute meanings and motives without checking them out first. For example:

If your partner doesn't make the first move, you may assume a loss of sexual interest or attraction. But it could also be that your partner doesn't want to cause physical injury and is being overly cautious while waiting for you to take the initiative.

Conversely, if your partner does make the first move, you may assume he is only interested in sex and not in your total well-being. But it could also be that your partner wants to build up your confidence and reassure you that he still loves you and finds you appealing. Perhaps he doesn't know how else to get the message across.

You can avoid the anxiety and pressure associated with resuming sexual activity by taking the initiative. Either make the first move or give your partner a clear signal that says "I'm ready for *you* to make the first move." After all, your partner isn't a mind reader, and you're the only one who really knows when you're feeling ready to resume sexual activity.

Summary

There are two categories of problems we experience as breast cancer patients: unavoidable and avoidable.

Unavoidable problems are universal. They are innate and affect each of us in similar ways. Although unavoidable, they are controllable.

Avoidable problems are manufactured. They are not innate. They occur when someone unintentionally says or does something that hurts us and we fail to speak up.

The way we respond to other people determines whether we will prevent or experience avoidable problems.

In order to steer clear of avoidable problems, we must first be in touch with how and what we are feeling.

If it's too late to *avoid* a problem, we can learn to *repair* it.

Becoming aware of potential avoidable problems can help us to prevent them and reduce our stress level.

We have complete control over the avoidable problems if we so choose.

Examples of avoidable problems that can occur during diagnosis include:
- agreeing to a one-step procedure
- seeking second opinions from doctors who aren't breast cancer specialists

Examples of avoidable problems that can occur during treatment include:
- failing to get written information about physical side effects
- scheduling appointments that are difficult to keep

Examples of avoidable problems that can occur during recovery include:
- Following someone else's timetable
- Expectations about resuming sexual activity

CHAPTER TWO

The Patient-
Doctor
Relationship

*T*he first and best place to find avoidable problems in action is in the patient-doctor relationship. Let's see how they get started and what we can do to prevent them so that we can save ourselves a lot of unnecessary emotional anguish.

We know it is important to form a good patient-doctor relationship at the very beginning of our breast cancer odyssey. But how do you define "good"? What's good for one woman may be not-so-good for another.

For example, some of us want the cold, hard truth about our diagnosis, treatment, and prognosis. No beating around the bush, no mincing words, just get to the bottom line. Others of us would be horrified by such blunt, terse words from our doctors and would prefer a little more (or a lot more) time and hand-holding to help us digest all of this information. Still others of us would rather not deal at all with the stress of statistics and dry facts while we are in the midst of doing our damnedest to fight off the disease.

The point I'm getting at is this: In order to find the patient-doctor relationship that is right for you, you will need to be candid with yourself about how much you want to know about your breast cancer—Everything? Nothing? Something in-between?

How do you relate to authority figures? How do you want them to relate to you? Do you prefer a protective parent-child relationship to an equal-partners relationship?

Basically, there are three types of patient-doctor relationships—*traditional, liberated,* and *pioneering.* Psychologically, each has its pros and cons. Depending on how you see yourself and perceive your needs, you will find that you fit more comfortably into one model or type than the other.

The Traditional Relationship

The traditional relationship is the most typical and frequently experienced patient-doctor relationship. In this model, the physician (usually a male) is perceived as the benevolent father who keeps in mind his daughter's best interests when recommending treatment. The patient is the compliant daughter who may or may not agree with Dad's decisions, but dutifully follows his plan. Is there any woman on the planet earth who hasn't experienced this type of relationship with her doctor?

What are the emotional gains and losses in this relationship? This is a perfectly acceptable, viable patient-doctor relationship provided you are genuinely comfortable in the role of passive patient. Clearly, if you are an assertive individual or have leanings in that direction, this is neither suitable nor appropriate. Oh sure, it can be worked through and resolved over time, but why go out of your way to look for trouble when you already have more than enough for a story plot on a soap opera?

The traditional relationship works best for those of us

who tend to be conventional in our values and attitudes. Elaine is just such a patient.

> ELAINE is an attractive fifty-five-year-old woman who spent all of her adult life as a wife and mother. She enjoyed being a homemaker and raising children. She loved her husband, who, like her father, was the benevolent boss of the family. Since his decisions were generally wise and thoughtful, both at home and in business, there was never any need to question or discuss matters.
>
> When Elaine was diagnosed with breast cancer, her husband and the surgeon discussed the problem while Elaine sat and primarily listened. She had little desire to participate and was relieved when the two men arrived at the treatment decisions.

In order to determine whether a traditional relationship will work for you, ask yourself these questions: Do I prefer a nonassertive role in my relationships with authority figures? Am I more comfortable when I delegate important decision-making to the men in my life—be it father, husband, boyfriend, or boss? If the answers are yes, this model will work for you.

The upside is that:
• The treatment decision is left to your doctor. You are free of the overwhelming burden and responsibility of weighing the treatment options with their physical and psychological pros and cons.

• You have a knowledgeable, capable, and caring person in charge of your breast cancer.

But the downside is:
• Unilateral decisions rarely take into account your personal feelings. In other words, since you are a passive participant, it is difficult, if not impossible, for your doctor to know what impact these decisions will have (or are having) on your life.

This model frequently minimizes the importance of the emotional/psychological aspects of diagnosis, treatment,

and recovery. Therefore, you will have to be on your toes
when it comes to monitoring your emotional stability. If
you find that you are not coping as well as you expected,
it is imperative that you tell your doctor. He needs to know
this. Sometimes we don't want to admit to our doctors that
we are having a bad time because we are afraid they will
take it as a personal criticism. And there are those of us
who are reluctant to speak up because we don't want to be
seen as complainers or troublemakers.

Believe me, your doctor will not respond negatively to
your disclosure. Rather, he will help you get the support
and information you need either by providing it himself,
through his staff or a referral to a psychotherapist. Many
of my patients are in traditional patient-doctor relationships. Their physicians made the referral as soon as the
women spoke up and said they were going through difficult times.

• If you are unhappy with the outcome of your doctor's
decisions, there is a tendency to blame yourself for not
speaking up sooner, as well as to feel that the doctor
betrayed and failed you. This is especially true for women
who had mastectomies and later discovered they were
appropriate candidates for lumpectomy/radiation treatment but were never advised or encouraged in this direction.

The paternalistic style of the traditional relationship
rankles many women and brings us to the second basic
type of patient-doctor relationship: liberated.

The Liberated Relationship

The liberated relationship is one in which the patient
and doctor are equal partners in all decisions. This model
appears to be the wave of the future, due in large part to
consumer advocacy and the growing awareness of patients'
rights. Not surprisingly, patients tend to be a bit more
enthusiastic than physicians about these new shifts and
changes in the patient-doctor roles. Although some doc-

tors may initially resist offering a liberated type of relationship to their patients, I have never met any who refused to participate on an equal basis when the patient pressed the issue.

I could devote an entire book on why some doctors are resistant to the liberated type of patient-doctor relationship, but suffice it to say that it goes back to medical school training. Younger doctors seem to be more receptive to democratic decision-making.

Is a liberated relationship an emotionally healthy one? Only if you are willing to spend substantial time doing your homework. This means reading current material on breast cancer, seeking second opinions from various specialists in the field, and accepting your share of the responsibility for all decisions, regardless of outcome.

JUDY's motivation to pursue a liberated relationship was based on two significant facts. First, there was a history of breast cancer in her family that had sensitized her to what she would and would not accept in a patient-doctor relationship, should she ever be diagnosed herself. Second, she was a newspaper reporter and very used to pursuing people and investigating facts. When the diagnosis came she was not surprised, but of course she was very distraught. The surgeon who performed the biopsy balked at an equal-partners relationship and then finally agreed to it. Fran decided she didn't want any favors from him and began to search out the possibility of forming a healthier relationship elsewhere.

Within a week she found a team of specialists who encouraged her active participation and involvement. But what a week that was! She felt like there weren't enough hours in the day to meet and talk with everyone. And she wasn't sure if choosing a new team was such a good idea after all. However, once she got past that week of anxiety and uncertainty, she felt more in control of her life and her treatment. And she felt she had made the right decision.

As you can see, the liberated relationship is a tough one to establish if you have never done it before. Many of us are not used to being assertive in any of our relationships with authority figures, much less with our doctors. It requires a great deal of tenacity. Sometimes we have to get downright insistent and ornery. It's easy to get discouraged, say "To hell with it," and go for a more traditional relationship.

I see many of my patients struggle with the choice of traditioal vs. liberated patient-doctor relationship. And so did I. Experience and observation lead me to conclude that the traditional relationship can be very comforting during the diagnosis, treatment, and early phases of recovery when we are still experiencing shock and denial. However, with the passage of time, the traditional relationship does not wear as well as the liberated one. Why? After the smoke clears and the dust settles, we may find ourselves questioning whether we would have made the same choices and decisions that our doctors made on our behalf. When the answer is yes, we are at peace with ourselves. But when the answer is no, we have sailed into dark and emotionally turbulent waters.

What are the pros and cons of the liberated relationship?

Here's the upside:
• When we actively participate in the treatment decisions we feel more in control, less helpless, and more willing to accept the outcome and results of these decisions.

And now for the downside:
• Initially, there are high levels of stress and anxiety due to the copious amounts of information bombarding us at once—and these decisions must be made within a relatively brief time span.

The Pioneering Patient-Doctor Relationship

Somewhere to the left of the liberated relationship is the pioneer. This relationship is unusual and does not apply to most of us. Essentially, you participate as a patient in an approved medical study (called a "clinical trial"), conducted by reputable physicians in a research hospital, such as the National Cancer Institute in Bethesda, Maryland. In this study, two or more methods for treating breast cancer are compared to determine if one is more effective than the other in controlling the cancer and achieving long-term survival. Your participation includes random assignment to one of the treatment groups. In other words, you have no say over which treatment you wind up with. However, if you are unhappy with the luck of the draw, you are under no obligation to remain in the study, and may go elsewhere for treatment.

Why would anyone choose this type of relationship over traditional or liberated? One big reason is financial. As you probably already know, breast cancer treatment is expensive. And state-of-the-art breast cancer treatment is outrageously expensive. Health insurance rarely covers the full cost. Many of us do not have adequate health insurance coverage, and some of us have no health insurance whatsoever. Health insurance concerns are covered in Chapter Five ("Getting Professional Help: Sooner Is Better") and Chapter Eight ("Getting Back to Business: Career and Job Issues"). Clinical trials offer patients with limited funds free and/or low-fee breast cancer treatment, including transportation, and room and board (if you live far away). Some even offer free psychological evaluation and psychotherapy. Pioneering spirit is admirable and without it, few advances would be made in the treatment of breast cancer.

The advantages are:

1. The financial cost is little or none.

2. The treatment is frequently one step ahead of state-of-the-art treatment.

3. You become a very important and special patient to your team of doctors. (Is there any breast cancer patient who hasn't had that wish? I can't even count the number of times that thought crossed my mind during the course of my treatment.)

But there can be disadvantages:

1. Is it worth your time? You may be required to travel a greater distance for your treatment than you would if you stayed closer to home. Also, the schedule of appointments may not be as convenient.

2. The emotional wear and tear may not be worth the money saved.

3. Of greatest concern—if the treatment fails, you may have unnecessarily jeopardized your breast and possibly your life.

The Unorthodox/Experimental Relationship

Frequently confused with the pioneering relationship is the unorthodox/experimental relationship. *Run* from any "doctor" who offers you a "miracle" drug, food, vitamin, or psychotherapy that will cure you. While there is growing evidence that mind-body interaction, good nutrition, vitamins, relaxation, and stress reduction can play a helpful role in your treatment plan, there is no scientific evidence that any of these treatments *alone* can cure breast cancer.

Why do some of us seek out unorthodox relationships and unproven treatment?

1. Promises from a quack may sound more appealing than the facts from a physician.

2. If we know someone who wasn't cured with conventional treatment, we may fear the same fate for ourselves.

3. We may have heard war stories about conventional treatment side effects, which are scary and intimidating.

If you feel you must enter into this type of relationship and treatment, do it *in addition to* (not instead of) a conventional relationship and treatment.

What if we are in a traditional relationship and we want to switch to a liberated one or vice versa? Is it too late? No! It's never too late to have the kind of patient-doctor relationship that is comfortable for each of us. But please remember that our doctors aren't mind readers, and we need to inform them of our decisions since we will need their cooperation and participation.

In addition to the type of patient-doctor relationship we will have (which is essentially a personal preference and not a matter of right or wrong), there are even more fundamental issues to be considered when selecting our doctors. I call them the ABC's—availability, bedside manner, and competence.

I have compiled a list of questions to ask. Carefully consider the answers *before* choosing your general surgeon, oncologist, reconstructive surgeon and/or radiation oncologist.

Availability

1. How available is this doctor—geographically, physically, and emotionally? Is his office within reasonable travel distance? If you need to stay overnight, do you have the time and money? Does he have regular and convenient office hours? Is he genuinely interested in having you as a

patient or do you have the feeling that he is overbooked and too busy to see you?

2. Does he return your phone calls? The same day?

3. Does he set aside enough time for you to ask questions at the end of each visit? Does he encourage you to ask questions?

4. Is he planning an extended vacation or absence during your treatment that will necessitate your seeing another doctor?

Some breast cancer specialists are so tuned-in to the availability issues that they work evenings, weekends, and holidays when necessary. One of my favorite doctors received an emergency phone call at 6 P.M. on July 3 from a woman he had never met who had just been diagnosed. She was frightened and needed reassurance as well as a consultation about treatment options. Although the doctor was looking forward to a relaxing Fourth of July weekend with his family, he talked with her at length and then the following morning he met with her in his office for a full consultation. From my perspective, this is a doctor who truly understands what it means to "be there" for his patients.

Even though it is not always possible for our doctors to be available to us, some are solving the problem in an innovative way. They work with a "patient educator" who functions as a liaison between patient and doctor, answering questions and providing written and verbal information. When there is a special request, problem, or concern that the patient educator cannot handle, a meeting is set up between the patient and doctor. Most patients are satisfied with this arrangement because they know that someone who is knowledgeable, caring, and officially endorsed by the doctor is always available to answer questions, dispense accurate information, and trouble-shoot when necessary.

Bedside Manner

Some may argue that bedside manner is a question of personal taste and style, but I feel there are certain basics you are entitled to and should look for:

1. Is he pleasant when he examines and talks to you?

2. Is he interested in what you have to say?

3. Is he sensitive to your feelings?

4. Does he encourage you to express your thoughts and feelings?

5. Does he provide thoughtful and understandable answers to your questions?

6. Is he tactful and diplomatic?

7. Is he prompt?

8. Does he refrain from taking phone calls during your examination and conference? If yes, will he honor that courtesy if you decide to become his patient? (Don't take it for granted, tell him it's important to you!)

I'm sorry to say that far too many breast cancer specialists have little or no bedside manner and don't even realize it. One of the top doctors in Los Angeles has an annoying habit of taking telephone calls from patients while he is in consultation with another. Not only is this rude to the patient sitting in his office, but consider the poor woman on the phone who thinks she is having a private and confidential conversation with her doctor!

I suppose if I were giving an Academy Award for "Most Devastating Bedside Manner," there would be a tie for first place between:

• the gynecologist who invited the patient into his office, informed her that she had breast cancer, and before she could respond, asked her to step into the waiting room while he answered a telephone call. (I promise this is true. I was seated in the waiting room when the stunned patient emerged.)

• the surgeon who telephoned the patient regarding her breast biopsy results. He cheerfully began, "I have good new and bad news. The bad news is you have breast cancer. The good news is yours is the best kind to get." The bewildered patient responded, "Is this some kind of joke?"

There is a lesson to be learned. A diagnosis of breast cancer deserves and demands your doctor's full and undivided attention—in person, not over the telephone, and without interruption. No patient should ever have to settle for anything less.

Bedside manner can make or break the patient-doctor relationship more than any of us may realize.

GLENDA was several months into her chemotherapy treatment and very unhappy. The oncologist never conversed with her and when she asked questions, he responded with yes/no answers. She concluded (erroneously) that the doctor was hiding something from her, she was receiving incorrect treatment, and that her condition had worsened or was not responding to treatment. Rather than worry and wonder, her anxiety motivated her to get a second opinion.

She consulted with an oncologist who I knew to be a friendly, chatty fellow. He reassured her that her fears were unfounded and that everything was A-OK. But he sensed correctly that she needed some TLC and hand holding. So he spent two hours talking with her and allaying her concerns. Guess what happened? Glenda was so thrilled to find an oncologist who willingly and unbegrudgingly conversed with her that she stayed with him and completed the same treatment she had begun elsewhere.

Conclusion? It is not impossible to find doctors who have a caring and gentle bedside manner. But we may have to look around a little longer for them.

Competence

1. What is this doctor's reputation within the medical community? (Ask several physicians you trust and with whom you have good rapport. Informed friends may be a good source for referrals too.)

2. Does this doctor specialize in treating breast cancer? How many breast cancer cases has he treated this year? Last year? How about checking his credentials? Try *The Directory of Medical Specialists,* a reference book that is updated every two years and is available in your local public library.

3. Is the doctor offering you experimental or unproven forms of treatment in lieu of mainstream medicine? Why?

4. Is this doctor practicing in a large city and on staff at a major, city, or regional hospital? I know this may sound snobbish, but trust me. When it comes to breast cancer, the movers and shakers go to the big cities . . . and so should you. I'm not knocking small-town doctors. They

are fine for uncomplicated illnesses, but not for up-to-date breast cancer treatment, where multimillion-dollar equipment is required that is cost-prohibitive in small-town hospitals.

When it comes to competence, I don't subscribe to the notion of a little or a lot. It's like being pregnant. You either *are* or you *aren't*. There is also no individual breast cancer specialist who is "the best." Remember when you were a little girl and your mother told you "There's more than one fish in the sea"? Well, the same is true about competent breast cancer specialists. There's more than one in every large city.

Listing the ABC's in order of importance, I put competence at the top, followed by availability. Bedside manner is not to be minimized, but it is definitely in third place, which is lucky for patient and doctor alike since it is in such short supply. Perhaps one day medical training for breast cancer will include serious course work and internships that are devoted to the psychological aspects of the patient-doctor relationship.

Before I get carried away with what physicians ought to do to improve the patient-doctor relationship, let's take a look at what we ourselves can do to improve the patient-doctor relationship.

1. Be prompt. If you want/expect your doctor to respect your time commitments, you must be willing to respect his.

2. Try not to cancel. Apart from the fact that cancellations, especially at the last minute, are usually annoying because they leave a big hole in the doctor's appointment schedule (and are not likely to increase your popularity with the nurses, technicians, and office staff), you may also wind up sabotaging your own treatment. Certain procedures are on timed schedules or doses (chemother-

apy, radiation, some surgical procedures) and you may be compromising your own prognosis and health. A good rule of thumb is this—don't cancel unless you are too sick to crawl out of bed. And frankly, if you're *that* sick, you *need* to be seen!

3. If you have several questions or wish extra time to speak with your doctor, tell the front desk when you set up the appointment. You will be given a time that is mutually convenient for both of you. Don't wait until the day of your appointment to request extra time. In all probability you won't get it because the schedule will be full. You will be disappointed and feel unnecessarily rejected.

4. Write down your questions ahead of time rather than trying to retrieve them from memory while you are talking with the doctor. If you don't, it's a cinch that you will forget them and then remember what you forgot just as soon as you leave the doctor's office.

5. Take notes and write down the answers to your questions. Better still, ask permission to bring a small cassette recorder with you whenever you have meetings with your doctors. This will help you process and digest new information that may be confusing and subject to distortions and erroneous recall. At the same time, it will save you many anxious hours and sleepless nights of wondering whether you are accurately remembering what was said.

6. Be direct in your communications. If you have a request, a problem, or a complaint, let your doctor know so that it can be resolved right away. Most physicians value your feedback and are genuinely interested in improving their services and meeting their patients' needs, but we have to let them know. Unfortunately, many of us insist on playing the role of the perfect patient who never com-

plains and is always nice. I'm not suggesting that you become nasty, but if you are unhappy with your doctor, his staff, the treatment, and/or anything else that is breast cancer–related, you owe it to yourself and your emotional well-being to make your concerns heard.

7. Follow the doctor's instructions. Don't improvise. If the instructions seem unreasonable, check to make sure you understood them correctly and discuss the possibility of modification or change. For example, if you are told not to drive for two weeks following breast surgery and axillary node dissection, and you feel up to driving within a week, get the medical okay before you take matters into your own hands. Without it you may be compromising your treatment and cosmetic results, as well as irritating the doctor, who may begin to see you as a difficult patient.

A difficult patient is one who creates unnecessary problems that complicate treatment and/or recovery, and are time-consuming to the physician and staff. Please be reassured that one misunderstanding will not earn you the reputation of being a difficult patient. But certainly habitual and chronic disregard for instructions will. For instance, if your doctor tells you it will take six to eight weeks before you can safely return to work, it is pointless to call his office every few days to report that you feel fine and wonder if he has changed his mind. Why not use the time constructively to give yourself a special treat—like going to museums, art galleries, concerts, catching up on your reading or movies you've missed? Physicians call it "patient compliance" and patients call it "following doctor's orders." One reason some of us find it a problem is that we tend to feel so controlled by our doctors and/or breast cancer that we grasp (sometimes mistakenly) for any little bit of power that will prove to ourselves and our doctors that we are not helpless. Rushing back to work and driving prematurely are two cases in point.

8. Be businesslike with your bill payments and with your health insurance refunds. If your company mistakenly sends the reimbursement check to you instead of your physician, present the check immediately to your doctor's office. Do not cash the check and later feign ignorance, confusion, or stupidity when you are found out. And I promise that you *will* be found out and will be plenty embarrassed too! Also, unless you have been advised to the contrary, you are expected to pay for whatever your insurance does not cover.

9. Your doctor is only human. Avoid placing him on a pedestal. Once there, the only place to go is down . . . and with a thud! The main problem with idealizing your doctor is he cannot possibly live up to your expectations and fantasies. Once the bubble bursts, you are apt to feel disappointed, angry, and anxious to switch physicians. And if you do switch, you are likely to repeat the same pattern all over again.

Even in the best patient-doctor relationships, there are awkward, embarrassing, and comical situations. For example, everyone knows that it is common to become infatuated with your doctor . . . especially when he has saved your life. While it's happening, it feels like love. A year later, you will recognize it for what it was and will chuckle to yourself about it.

Another awkward situation is the fear/belief that your doctor has made a mistake or isn't giving you the right treatment. This is a universal fear that each of us experiences at some point. I'm not talking about the initial reaction of "Not me . . . there must be some mistake." I'm referring to a wave of panic that washes over you at the moment you decide a serious and irreversible error has been made. Here's one of the beauties I pulled: During my third week of radiation therapy, I became convinced that my head was not in the proper position for several of the treatments and, consequently, my brain was accidentally fried. No one could convince me otherwise.

When these panicky thoughts hit you, two questions to ask yourself are: 1) Why am I having these thoughts *now?* (Usually we are upset at something or someone else, and without realizing it we grab onto the most convenient target.) 2) What can I do to alleviate my panic? If you are certain you are not upset with someone else and are not displacing your feelings onto your doctor or your treatment, then the healthiest and smartest course of action is to present your concerns to the doctor. This will give both of you a chance to examine the reality of the situation.

There is no point in keeping your fears to yourself as it will only upset you and cause distance and mistrust in the patient-doctor relationship.

There is also no point in seeking a second opinion without first discussing the problem with the doctor who is treating you. Why? Because doctor #2 will need your records from doctor #1 in order to intelligently assess your diagnosis and treatment. In other words, doctor #1 is going to find out anyway, so why not give him the courtesy of finding out from you?

How does this affect the relationship? Frankly, I have never known a competent doctor who insisted on talking the patient out of a second opinion. I'm not saying that they love it, either. They don't. It's a big red flag that something is wrong in the relationship. Sometimes it isn't treatment competency at all, but rather the availability or bedside manner, or a communication breakdown that is at the root of the problem.

In any case, you are not the first patient to feel that your doctor has made an error, nor will you be the last. Doctors expect it. It comes with the territory. So take a deep breath, talk to doctor #1 and then, for your own peace of mind, talk to doctor #2 as well. You will sleep better for it. And if it turns out that it was all in your imagination, don't feel bad. Welcome to the club!

One of the ways that each of us defends against the fear and anger of having breast cancer is to blame the doctor for making mistakes. Sometimes it's real, sometimes it's imagined. That's why it is so important to talk with him before we run elsewhere or threaten a malpractice suit. Speaking of which . . .

The only sure-fire way that I know to ruin a patient-doctor relationship is to threaten and/or implement a malpractice lawsuit. Obviously, if your grievance is legitimate, this should not be a deterrent. But if there is any doubt in your mind, then please do yourself a favor and consider the following repercussions prior to taking verbal or legal action:

1. If the medical community feels there is even a shadow of doubt as to blame, it will be tough finding a breast cancer specialist who will be willing to testify against your doctor. (The operative sentiments seem to be "Let he who is without sin cast the first stone" and "There but for the grace of God go I.")

2. Win or lose, you may find it difficult (if not impossible) to ever receive follow-up breast cancer care in that community. Is this right, fair, ethical, or moral? Of course not. But it is a reality and one that you will have to live with if you decide to walk down this path.

Although it is highly unlikely that you will be in need of filing a malpractice suit, my purpose in discussing this issue is to point out how important it is to screen your doctors carefully and thoroughly *before* you begin treatment instead of living with litigation after the fact.

We have seen how the patient-doctor relationship can increase or decrease our fantasies and fears about our breast cancer. Much of what we feel about our disease depends on the kind of relationship we have with our doctors and their attitudes toward treatment and us. In other words, we have a lot of control over the avoidable problems and, in turn, over our emotional well-being simply by choosing competent doctors with whom we are comfortable and who relate to us in a way that puts us at ease.

Summary

There are three types of patient-doctor relationships: traditional, liberated, pioneer. Each has its pros and cons.

The ABC's of choosing your team of doctors are: Availability, Bedside Manner, and Competence.

Fifty percent of the patient-doctor relationship depends on the patient. Our attitudes and behavior can either help or hinder the relationship and, in turn, our treatment experience.

Awkward and embarrassing moments are inevitable, and run the gamut of developing a schoolgirl crush on your doctor to thinking that he has made a serious error in your treatment.

The surest way to ruin the patient-doctor relationship is to threaten/file a malpractice suit. So carefully screen your doctors *before* treatment instead of living with regret *after*.

CHAPTER THREE

Adjusting

to the

Diagnosis

*R*eceiving the diagnosis of breast cancer is an emotionally devastating experience. Anyone who tells you otherwise hasn't had the disease.

What makes this diagnosis so traumatic? The fact that no one is ever psychologically prepared for the blow (not even those of us who have a history of breast cancer in the family). It is for this reason many women find adjusting to the diagnosis more difficult than coping with the treatment itself.

The range of reactions and feelings paint a vivid picture of the first moment of truth:

"I felt like I had been flattened by a steamroller."

"A bad nightmare that I couldn't wake up from . . ."

"I got nauseous . . . felt like I was going to throw up on myself . . ."

". . . like a knot in the pit of my stomach . . ."

"I was too numb to hear and too shocked to speak."

"My mind left my body. I was watching this other woman
and my doctor talk. It was happening to someone else,
someone who vaguely resembled me. I saw her break into
a million little pieces before my very eyes."

Show me a woman who doesn't have a strong reaction to
the diagnosis and I'll show you a woman in a coma.
Nevertheless, many of us try to hide or minimize our
initial reactions from our doctors, family, friends, and,
worst of all, from ourselves.

Consider the irony: When we are diagnosed with
chicken pox or the measles, we bemoan our condition, feel
sorry for ourselves, and expect lots of comfort and support. But when we are diagnosed with breast cancer, we
quietly slink into a corner hoping no one will notice us or
find out about our condition. Is this supposed to make us
feel better? If so, it doesn't work very well since most of us
wind up feeling worse. Does hiding or remaining silent
make any sense? Of course not. We are not criminals on
the lam! For our own sanity and well-being, we need to
stop doing this to ourselves.

Our fears need to be expressed and heard. When we
swallow our feelings we make our overall adjustment to
the diagnosis even more difficult, lonely, and painful. In
some instances, we actually scare ourselves away from
receiving treatment.

Ready or not, the diagnosis propels us into a crisis state
that is universal and unavoidable. We experience shock,
disbelief, confusion, fear, horror, panic, denial, anger,
grief, and more—but not necessarily in that order. I have
known women to experience all of these reactions within a
ten-minute time span! For others it takes hours, days, and
even weeks of mood swings back and forth from one
intense feeling to the next. Ultimately, we are worn out by
our emotions and we reach the point of exhaustion and
acceptance.

Is it abnormal to experience these mood changes and

outbursts? No! They are a normal, expected part of the process of coping with the diagnosis. In fact, it would be extremely unusual if you didn't experience this. It is unhealthy to keep our feelings bound up inside. It leads to serious depression later on—usually during recovery.

Our willingness to express our initial feelings is necessary, therapeutic, and says a lot about how we will cope with the entire breast cancer odyssey. With this in mind, it shouldn't surprise you to find out that *crybabies cope better than strong, silent types.* So when your friends ask what they can do for you during this time, tell them to bring over a big box of tissues and a comfortable shoulder to cry on.

Speaking of crying, I would like to dispel the popular notion that a little bit of crying is good, but a lot is bad. First of all, whose measuring cup are we using? What amounts to a lot of tears for one woman may be not enough for another. Second, what is there to be gained by holding back tears? It doesn't make you a better person. It just makes you depressed.

Crying is a constructive way to ventilate your feelings when you are adjusting to the diagnosis. The only time it is harmful or dangerous is when you are driving and can't see the car in front of you. Crying releases tensions and stress. As does pounding pillows and mattresses with your fists. So the next time someone advises, "It's not good to cry too much," ask them, "Who isn't it good for, me or you?"

What are the major pitfalls that prevent us from making a healthy adjustment to the diagnosis?

Denial

Like exotic perfume, a little denial goes a long way. All of us use denial to some extent, not only to help us adjust to the diagnosis of breast cancer, but to help us adjust to life! There are four classic styles:

1. *The Runaway:* Some of us get so shocked and scared that we insist the diagnosis isn't true. We refuse to acknowledge our feelings or ventilate them to ourselves or anyone else. Instead, we bolt for the door and are never seen or heard from again. Obviously, the breast cancer doesn't go away just because we do. Is there anything to be gained by running? Nothing. Wherever you go, you take yourself and your diagnosis with you.

Is there any one of us who can honestly say that she didn't consider—at least for one brief moment—running away from the diagnosis? Let's admit it, it's a gut reaction that is universal and unavoidable. Even though we have the impulse to flee, we don't have to act on it. We can *gain control* over the feeling by *talking* about it. Fortunately, that's what most of us do.

2. *The Pollyanna:* This is when we adjust so well and so quickly that it's just too good to be true. In this instance, we cheerfully accept the diagnosis as if it were happy news. We don't complain or express negative thoughts and feelings to others. In some extreme cases, we may actually find ourselves saying to family and friends that this was the best thing that ever happened to us!!! But deep within our hearts, we know it's a lie. In fact, the diagnosis has thrown us into a frightening emotional tailspin and we are too ashamed to admit or express our feelings to anyone except ourselves.

There is a touch of Pollyanna in all of us . . . the need to feign serenity in the face of disaster, in order to make others believe we are in better shape than we actually are. It's a universal/unavoidable feeling. But we don't have to become a victim. We can gain control by expressing the feelings verbally.

3. *Wonder Woman:* If you are a career woman or a professional, you may recognize Wonder Woman in yourself. Typically, we become stoic, strong, emotionless, and *overly controlled.* Although intellectually we are willing to acknowledge to ourselves and others that we are "concerned" (we would never use the word "afraid"), we refuse to express these feelings to anyone including ourselves. We keep all of our feelings bottled up until the cork is ready to pop. And when it pops, and it always does, we rapidly advance into a closet case.

4. *The Closet Case:* Like Clark Kent's clone, we are Wonder Woman by day and merely mortal by night. In the privacy of her own home, when no one is watching, the closet case allows the floodgates to open and the emotions to come pouring out. While it is good that the feelings are being ventilated, it is sad that we feel they must be kept hidden all day.

Which of the four types best describes you? Some of us are a combination—one type during diagnosis, another type during treatment and recovery. Don't worry, it's okay for you to see yourself in these four denial styles. After all, none of us will ever change the denial behavior unless we first acknowledge its existence. Besides, who's kidding whom? It takes one to know one. Aren't we all in this boat together?

Incidentally, high intelligence has nothing to do with ability to express feelings or make a healthy adjustment to the diagnosis. Some of the smartest women have made some of the biggest blunders.

MARCY was a successful stockbroker who graduated Phi Beta Kappa from a top Eastern school of business. She was so intimidated by the diagnosis of breast cancer that she decided to tell no one . . . including her boyfriend. She was afraid that he would leave her once he found out. So she picked a fight and broke up with him first. Did this help her to feel better? Of course not. It helped her to feel worse—more alone and trapped. Fortunately, she was aware enough to realize what a giant goof she had made before the relationship became history.

The second major pitfall in adjusting to the diagnosis is:

Guilt

Some of us feel we have only ourselves to blame for the diagnosis of breast cancer. We didn't measure up as human beings and, therefore, we got what we deserved. Perhaps we believe we weren't sufficiently giving, loving, or good enough. Or maybe we didn't follow the proper health regimen regarding diet, exercise, and sleep.

If guilt is your hobby, you can come up with more than a hundred creative ways to torture and convince yourself that you brought this upon yourself. Although I can't stop you from this train of thought, I strongly recommend you consider a more cheerful form of recreation.

And for the record: Is there any scientific evidence that guilt causes breast cancer? No. How about that breast cancer is a punishment for some prior misdeed or infraction? No. Are there certain activities, thoughts, or feelings that promote/prevent breast cancer—like sex, for instance? No. Does guilt serve any useful purpose in trying to adjust to the diagnosis. No. (Nor does it serve any useful purpose during treatment or recovery.)

No one knows what causes breast cancer. When the cause is discovered, it won't be kept secret. We will certainly hear about it in the news media. However, we do know what causes guilt: poor self-image and low self-worth. It's the "whatever goes wrong is my fault" syndrome. Instead of trying to build a case as to why you are to blame for your diagnosis, why not put your energy into building up your self-esteem?

Guilt feelings and reactions cause avoidable problems. They can be prevented or remedied by speaking up and setting the record straight—first with yourself, second with anyone who states or implies that you are in some way personally responsible for your diagnosis.

Stress

Stress is a hot topic these days. A surprising number of people believe that stress causes breast cancer. My response is this: Do you know any adult woman who hasn't experienced stress in her personal or professional life in the last year or two? No. Now ask yourself, how come they didn't get breast cancer and I did?

We all know that stress is not healthy. Many of us believe that it should be avoided because it lowers our immune system's resistance (physically and psychologically) to a wide range of illnesses, including the common cold. But to insist on a direct cause-and-effect relationship between stress and breast cancer defies the laws of logic since most women don't get breast cancer but all women experience stress.

There are two core issues that emerge during the process of adjusting to the diagnosis. Both are universal and unavoidable:

• The fear of dying.

• The fear of losing or changing the appearance of our breasts.

Many people have the mistaken notion that concern over breast appearance is trivial when compared to survival. Wanting to stay "whole" is far from trivial. No one wants to lose any part of the anatomy, especially one that is integral to feelings of being female and maternal. For many of us, the appearance of our breasts relates directly to the quality of our lives and our will to live. In this culture, such feelings are very understandable. And if these should be your feelings, you have no reason to apologize or justify your position. For better or worse, most of us are women whose attitudes were influenced by *Playboy* magazine and the emphasis on big, beautiful breasts.

What makes one woman choose "quality of life" while another opts for "quantity of life"? The psychological/emotional factors that influence these decisions will be discussed in Chapter Six ("The Psychological Effects of our Treatment Decisions"). For now, suffice it to say that many women feel that without quality of life, quantity is meaningless. And for some, quality is defined as having reasonably attractive breasts.

Now we may not all agree with that philosophical position, or with women who make that decision. Nevertheless, it is an understandable dilemma. It is yet another universal, unavoidable issue that each of us has wrestled with on at least one or more occasions. And for some of us, it is a real tug of war. Fortunately, the majority of us come to realize that quantity and quality of life don't have to be an either/or choice.

What factors determine how well each of us will handle the diagnosis?

1. *Who breaks the bad news.*
Is it a doctor with whom we have an established and

trusting relationship (such as our internist or gynecologist)? Or is it a doctor who is new to us? Ideally, the information should be presented by someone who knows us and with whom we have good rapport. But practically speaking, we will probably find out from the surgeon who performed the biopsy. In many instances, we have met the surgeon only once prior to the biopsy.

It is a very weird feeling when a relative stranger presents you with life-shattering news. Not surprisingly, the surgeon feels pretty uncomfortable too. There is almost nothing he can say or do to make the situation better, and just about anything can and will make it worse.

Some surgeons fear we will revert to the ancient Greek custom of killing the messenger who is the bearer of the bad news: in other words, that we will act as if the doctor caused the breast cancer, when he is only reporting the findings.

The decision as to which doctor breaks the news can get needlessly complicated and confusing:

> HALLIE discovered a lump in her breast and went to the gynecologist to have it checked. She was referred to a radiologist for a mammogram. Although the radiologist knew immediately from the X-ray that Hallie had breast cancer, he was reluctant to tell her. Instead, he advised that she return to her own doctor to get the results. Hallie was annoyed. She felt this was a roundabout way of getting the answer to a crucial question and that the doctors were being needlessly overprotective.

Were they or weren't they? It's hard to say. Some of us will gladly forgo rapport and intimacy in order to get the information quickly. We are anxious to find out the results as soon as possible. Others of us are in no great hurry and would prefer to wait a few hours or even a few days to get the full story from someone we know and trust.

Is one decision healthier than the other? No. It's a

matter of choice. And here is the important point—the choice should always be yours. Let your doctors know whether you prefer that all information be relayed first to your primary physician or whether the first communication of information should go directly to you. And don't wait to be asked first. This isn't a tea dance. It's your life. Volunteer your preferences. It makes for fewer misunderstandings and preventable problems all the way around.

2. *How the bad news is broken.*

You don't have to know much about breast cancer to know whether you feel *connected with* or *alienated from* the doctor who gives you the diagnosis. Is your doctor gentle or brusque? Leisurely or rushed? Concerned or indifferent?

It goes without saying that an in-person consultation with your doctor is highly desirable and that a hasty phone call that catches you off guard is an open invitation to problems.

IRIS couldn't understand why the doctor wanted her to return to his office to get the biopsy results. She was busy, and it seemed like a waste of time and money. She asked the doctor to telephone her instead. Reluctantly, the doctor agreed. It was a big mistake. Instead of the good news she expected, Iris received a diagnosis of breast cancer. It was late on a Friday afternoon, and she was alone, frightened, and too stunned to ask questions. She suffered through an agonizing weekend. On Monday, she went to the doctor's office and asked the questions that would have been answered several days earlier, had she met with her doctor in person.

Was this problem avoidable? Of course. Iris made a decision without thinking it through. Her doctor went along with it, which compounded the error. She gambled that it would turn out favorably. It didn't. She paid a high price for the convenience of a phone call. The inconvenience of an anxiety-filled weekend was certainly greater than the inconvenience of a follow-up visit. (Incidentally, most doctors don't charge an extra fee for a post-biopsy visit.)

Is there a lesson to be learned? I believe so. Physicians are busy people who don't insist on no-fee return visits that are trivial. A biopsy for breast cancer is important and worthy of a follow-up visit . . . even when the results are benign.

3. *Our prior experiences with breast cancer.*

Family History. If there is no family history of breast cancer, the initial reaction is typically one of shock and disbelief, followed by intense mood swings. Even when there is a family history, we may still feel a wide, gripping range of emotions. But in all likelihood we have already considered the possibilities of breast cancer occurring in our lives.

Does this mean that if we have a family history we will have a better emotional adjustment to the diagnosis? Yes and no. Yes, if our experience is that our mother, aunt, or other female relative went on to live a long and productive life following the diagnosis and treatment. No, if our experience is that the diagnosis marked the end of life, either physically, emotionally, or both.

While a family history can prepare you for a diagnosis, it certainly doesn't guarantee an easier adjustment.

JILL's mother died from advanced breast cancer. Her prognosis was poor because she was diagnosed too late to change the course of the illness. Many years later, Jill was diagnosed with an early breast cancer, and her prognosis was excellent. Nevertheless, Jill was fearful she would wind up sharing her mother's fate. With the help of bibliotherapy (reading materials such as books and pamphlets) as well as some individual psychotherapy, Jill was able to reduce her anxiety, accept that she was not her mother's twin, and realize that early detection had saved her own life (and it might well have saved her mother's life had she been diagnosed sooner).

Some of us with a strong family history live in such dread of the diagnosis that we opt for prophylactic (preventative) mastectomies with immediate reconstruction, simply to avoid multiple biopsies and what we believe is an inevitable diagnosis sometime in our future. For many women, it is like buying an insurance policy against breast cancer. Others insist it is too drastic and prefer a wait and see approach. Many breast cancer specialists share the same sentiments—pro and con. As you can see, this procedure is controversial and emotionally charged for both patient and physician. It needs to be carefully thought through over time and discussed with more than one doctor before making a final decision. Nevertheless, the ultimate decision should always be your own.

Myths and War Stories. Let's face it, breast cancer has a lousy reputation. Not that there is anything particularly good to say in its defense, except that some of the bad image is pure hype. For example, how many times have we heard (or had it implied) that a diagnosis of breast cancer means an automatic death sentence? Some still believe this is so, even though there is overwhelming evidence to the contrary. It's a myth, and like any other piece of alarming gossip, it perpetuates a life of its own filled with doubt, fear, and panic. This myth has been handed down from one generation to the next, scaring countless women away from seeking diagnosis and treatment, not to mention early detection.

A patient recently told me that whenever someone says that breast cancer is an automatic death sentence she responds: "If you want to get technical, so is life."

While myths perpetuate a vague and generalized fear

of death and dying, war stories generate a more specific anxiety based on real-life experiences.

A classic war story usually goes something like this: Someone we know relishes telling us a tale of terror that befalls her friend or neighbor with breast cancer. The patient-friend invariably suffers unspeakable indignities and torture, making death seem like a welcomed relief. But, of course, this never happens because the woman doesn't even have enough good fortune to up and die. You begin to get the feeling that if it weren't for bad luck, this woman would have no luck at all. You subsequently meet the patient-friend and discover that most of what you were told about her experience was pure fantasy created by the mind and mouth of the storyteller. If you know nothing about breast cancer, which one will stay in your mind—the war story or the reality? For many, I'm afraid it's the war story.

If, prior to your diagnosis, you have heard myths and war stories, it may make your adjustment to the diagnosis more difficult because you are anticipating experiences similar to the ones you were told about. I know it is hard to forget what you have heard, but please remember that unless you have firsthand experience that tells you otherwise, these stories remain nothing more than trashy gossip that belongs in the garbage.

When it comes to myths and war stories, my philosophy is this: "Believe half of what you see and none of what you hear."

Media Exposure. Lucky for us the media is consumer-oriented and has done a lot to dispel myths, war stories, and other pieces of false information regarding breast cancer. This means that, for the most part, TV, radio, magazines, and newspapers have been accurate, informed, and up-beat in their coverage of breast cancer developments. In fact, the media deserves a lot of credit for informing women that early detection of breast cancer can save their lives, as well as their breasts. For example, KATHY credits television for making her diagnosis less intimidating:

> "The week before I found out I had breast cancer, I watched a show where they said that, in many cases, you didn't have to lose your breast if they found the cancer early. So when my doctor gave me the diagnosis, as scared and confused as I was, I remembered the TV show and asked him about it. Sure enough, he didn't have to take my breast. I know that having that information beforehand made my reaction to the diagnosis less frightening."

4. *What is going on in the rest of your life.*

It only stands to reason that if life is treating you well, the adjustment to the diagnosis will be easier than if your life is filled with catastrophes. When your life is packed with one crisis after another, coping with the diagnosis may prove to be the proverbial straw that broke the camel's back. If that's your situation, don't despair. You can actually use the diagnosis to your advantage.

> LISA was working full time and going to nursing school. She supported her teenage sons and her alcoholic husband, who had difficulty holding down a job. Her father had recently suffered a heart attack and she was shuttling back and forth from his apartment each day, making sure he got proper food and rest. Lisa was frazzled and worn out. It took getting diagnosed with breast cancer to make her stop and realize how exhausted and angry she felt. She knew she couldn't continue to be the only responsible member of her household.
>
> Lisa used the diagnosis to take a stand with her husband. She insisted that he get professional help or move out. She asked the teenagers to get part-time jobs after school so that she could cut back on working full time while she was in school. She also arranged with her brother to take turns caring for their father.

In other words, Lisa used the diagnosis to take care of herself. For the first time in her life, she felt entitled to put herself first.

Some may call Lisa selfish, and some may call her smart. I vote for smart.

Like Lisa, you too can use the diagnosis to straighten out your life. Keep what works and get rid of what doesn't and never will. A diagnosis of breast cancer will put your life and priorities into sharp focus. Take advantage of it. It's one of the positives that can emerge from this unpleasant experience.

At the same time you receive the blow of your diagnosis, you will be advised of your treatment options. You may feel pressured to make a decision—not necessarily by your doctor, but by your own panic and need to be rid of "it." This is not the time for quick decision-making. Don't pressure yourself into making treatment decisions until you have fully digested the news of the diagnosis. This takes at least a few days, if not longer. Reading (bibliotherapy) is an excellent way to bind your anxiety while simultaneously receiving accurate information. Start reading pamphlets and easy-to-read material on the subject.

This is also the time to get love, nurturance and emotional support. In addition to reaching out to family and friends, ask your doctor for the names of breast cancer–support groups, and for a referral to a psychotherapist who specializes in treating breast cancer patients. Having names and phone numbers is like having a nice cup of chicken soup. It couldn't hurt!

Summary

What can we do to facilitate a healthy emotional adjustment to the diagnosis?

• Acknowledge to yourself that you feel fear, anger, and many other uncomfortable feelings.

• Express these initial reactions and feelings to your doctor and then to those family members and friends who will be of emotional support to you.

• Accept that wanting to run away from the diagnosis is a normal feeling and doesn't mean that you are going to do it.

• Quit trying to impress others with how well you are keeping it together. If you feel like you're falling apart, don't pretend you're doing fine.

• Stop blaming yourself and/or allowing others to blame you for causing the breast cancer diagnosis.

• Don't pressure yourself into making treatment decisions until you have fully digested the news of the diagnosis. This takes at least a few days, if not longer.

• Even if you feel that you can't concentrate, start reading small sections of books and pamphlets on the subject (bibliotherapy). It's an excellent way to reduce your anxiety while you are getting accurate information.

• Ask your doctor for the names of breast cancer–support groups and for a referral to a psychotherapist who specializes in treating breast cancer patients.

Choosing Personal

Support Systems:

Who to Reach Out to

and How to Do It

*T*he family members and friends we turn to for emotional support following our breast cancer diagnosis seem to fall into two groups:

• Those who become a valuable source of emotional support, love, and warmth.

• Those who exacerbate our anxieties and fears.

This chapter identifies the similarities and differences between the two groups and the pitfalls to watch out for. We will learn how to make more accurate and thoughtful choices when we reach out for support. In other words, we will become "constructively selective."

When animals are hurt they go off by themselves and lick their wounds until they get better. Human beings are just the opposite. We instinctively reach out to family and friends. Animals do not expect members of the flock or pack to attend to their needs. Humans, however, anticipate their loved ones will provide comfort, support, and stability. That's how it's supposed to be. But it doesn't always work that way.

Once we get over the shock of the diagnosis and start telling the people closest to us, we may discover that we have only one person, maybe two, who respond in a way that lives up to our expectations. The rest of the people, no matter how well-intentioned they may be, seem to disappoint us. Some in ways that would appear petty to others but are significant to us—like a flip remark or a forgotten phone call from a friend.

What's going on here? Is it us? Are we being unrealistic or overly demanding? Is it them? Are they too self-centered or emotionally incapable of giving of themselves? The answer is: It's both! Sometimes it's us, sometimes it's them, and sometimes it's a combination of the two. First, let's take a look at us.

This is a very vulnerable time for us. We are flooded with thoughts and feelings that are confusing and frightening. This has an effect on our decision-making abilities in all aspects of our life, especially in our personal relationships.

We wouldn't think of going to an empty bank account when we need cash. Yet we often make a beeline to a relative or friend who is emotionally bankrupt, expecting comfort and support.

Why do we do this to ourselves? The answer is: When we are in crisis, we tend to forget the reality of what is and, instead, go for what we wish it would be. This is particularly true if the person carries a title that implies long-term intimacy, such as "Mother" or "Daughter."

In most instances, it is not unrealistic to assume that "Mother" will make herself emotionally available to "Daughter" (and vice versa) during critical times. But it is not necessarily realistic to expect that "Mother" has the emotional capacity to be there in a *meaningful* way for her "Daughter."

NINA was divorced and lived alone in Los Angeles. Her mother lived with her second husband in Boston. The first person Nina called after she got the diagnosis was her mother. She momentarily forgot that her mother had not been particularly supportive or nurturing in the past, and now that she was getting older seemed a trifle unstable as well.

Predictably, upon hearing the news, her mother went into a crisis. Instead of turning to her husband for strength, she looked to Nina. She telephoned her daughter several times a day, asking for reassurance that everything was going to be okay. Nina grew increasingly irritated and anxious with each phone call.

Instead of soothing Nina's fears and anxieties, her mother was intensifying them. It was Mother who was getting support from Nina, instead of the other way around! Poor Nina was out in the cold, without a support system to call her own.

This is an unfortunate, but not unusual, scenario. Some of us have an uncanny ability to reach out to the wrong people (in this case, the least stable family member) and expect them to come through like champs. When they don't, *we* wind up feeling like chumps.

Granted, this vignette definitely qualifies as an unavoidable problem inasmuch as a family member said and did all the wrong things and was emotionally unavailable at a critical time. But didn't Nina contribute to this mishap (and aggravate her own distress even further) by reaching out to her mother when there was no history of nurturing between them?

When you look for support from people who have not supported you in the past, you need to examine what's going on inside your own head. To be perfectly frank, Nina was not such an innocent victim. She was a glutton for punishment.

How can we avoid making this mistake? In most instances, the person in question has repeatedly demon-

strated that she is unable to be helpful in a crisis. On some
unconscious level, we already know this but don't want to
recognize it. Unfortunately for Nina, it took a diagnosis of
breast cancer to confirm a painful truth that she had been
dodging for years. But who could blame her?

No one wants to believe that her mother (or daughter)
can't or won't be emotionally supportive during times of
trauma. And the same is true for husbands and lovers who
want to be emotionally supportive and don't know how, as
well as those who think they are, when in fact they aren't.

Sometimes the men who love us don't understand what
we need from them. (So what else is new?) What they think
is emotional support may feel like just the opposite to us.
For example:

> When ANGELA was diagnosed, she anticipated her hus-
> band, Jack, would be her main source of comfort and
> support. To her utter amazement, he asked her to post-
> pone the surgery for a month because he had an important
> business trip lined up. Angela was devastated by his
> thoughtlessness.
>
> After meeting with Angela, I asked Jack to come to my
> office for a consultation so that I could get a better grasp
> of what was going on with him, her, and their relationship.
> Jack revealed that the previous year he had rescued his
> business from financial ruin and was now on the verge of
> signing a big deal that would provide enough money for
> retirement.
>
> He didn't think his request was inconsiderate since the
> money was going to benefit both of them. He loved his
> wife, but couldn't pass up the deal of a lifetime.
>
> We reached a compromise. Jack postponed the trip by
> three days until Angela was out of surgery. She reached
> out to her grown children for primary emotional support,
> and Jack telephoned her each night from his hotel room.

What is there to say about this case? That when we're
battling breast cancer, our husbands should put business

aside to be with us? That goes without saying. Ideally, Angela's diagnosis should have taken precedence over Jack's anxiety about his business trip. No question about it. Yet, throughout their marriage, Jack had placed his business ahead of his relationship with his wife and children. Jack was either working late or on a business trip when most of the traumas and illnesses occurred at home. Angela didn't like this arrangement, but she never complained about it either.

So, given this kind of track record, what else could we have expected from Jack? This doesn't excuse his behavior. It only explains it. Angela must have known before she told Jack of the diagnosis that he was not going to be her primary source of comfort and support. Their history together attested to that.

If your family history indicates the same type of pattern as that of Angela and Jack, or Nina and her mother, it's not very likely to change just because you now have breast cancer. So why set yourself up for even more disappointment and aggravation when you can avoid it? You're not going to make a silk purse out of a sow's ear. At least not while you are trying to cope with breast cancer. Forget about *what ought to be* and go for *what is*. Reach out to family/friends who have been emotionally supportive and available to you all along.

Sometimes our expectations of others are realistic in terms of their ability to be there for us, but not as often or as much as we would like. Instead of accepting the limitations of the relationship, we up the ante and become critical and demanding. We actually wind up driving the person away, when our intention is to draw the person closer.

When PENNY told her sister of her breast cancer diagnosis, Rita canceled her vacation plans to be with her sibling. Every day, Rita drove Penny to and from her doctor appointments, cooked, cleaned, shopped, and made her sis-

ter's life as comfortable as possible. Each evening, Rita
returned home to be with her husband. This upset Penny,
who felt abandoned and alone. Her resentment built up to
the point that she told Rita if she didn't stay overnight, she
didn't want her help during the day. Rita was stunned by
Penny's "my way or no way" ultimatum, and was unable to
reason with her. Ultimately, she withdrew from the relationship and told Penny to call if she changed her mind.

I think most of us would agree that Penny's behavior
was unreasonable and her demands excessive. Everyone
has personal needs and a life that goes on irrespective of
our breast cancer. Rita's unavailability in the evening certainly didn't diminish her concern and love for her sister,
as evidenced by her presence during the day.

How could Penny have avoided this situation? She could
have discussed her needs and Rita's availability beforehand
so they could have agreed on a mutually convenient plan.
And she could have reached out to *several* family members/
friends who were willing to cooperate with one another in
setting up a schedule that was comfortable and workable
for everyone. The team concept eliminates the problem of
one person feeling overwhelmed with responsibility and
our feeling disappointed and hurt if this person fails to
live up to our expectations.

How can Penny repair the relationship? An apology to
her sister is in order. Specifically, she needs to acknowledge that she was way out of line with her demands.
Additionally, a more realistic plan is required. Penny needs
to set up a new schedule that allows for Rita's personal
needs as well as her own.

There is a very fine line between realistic expectations
and unrealistic demands. Sometimes it's hard to tell when
we have crossed over the line. Here's a rule of thumb: If
you have a general feeling of anger toward the people you
have reached out to, it is usually a clear sign that your

expectations were unrealistic, either in terms of your requests, the people you selected, or both.

Now that we know the pitfalls to watch for in ourselves, what potentially hazardous traits should we watch for in others?

Is this person "cancerphobic"?

Sometimes a close friend or relative will become icy and distant when we tell them we have breast cancer. In extreme cases, they may literally vanish from our lives, possibly resurfacing weeks, months, even years later. It hurts a lot because we know we have done nothing to warrant the desertion. It's also impossibly frustrating because it's so illogical and irrational.

SANDY and Terri were good friends and former college roommates. Sandy shared the diagnosis with Terri the night before she went in for her surgery. Sandy assumed Terri would call or visit her in the hospital.

Terri didn't call for two weeks. She claimed she was too busy, couldn't visit, but would call again when she had time. Sandy was upset by Terri's indifference and spoke to her about it, right then and there.

Terri confessed she was afraid to be near Sandy because she had negative associations with cancer, stemming from childhood memories of her grandmother. Because of this, Terri chose to bow out of their friendship. For many months, Sandy was hurt and angry. This eventually melted into sadness at Terri's inability to function as a caring, compassionate human being because she was so riddled with senseless fear.

What can we learn from Sandy's experience? When we reach out to those close to us, we need to find out how they feel about cancer in general and breast cancer in particular. If they get panicky or are unable to maintain the conversation, there's a good chance they are "cancer-phobic" (irrationally fearful of cancer and/or anything vaguely related). A true "breast cancerphobic" avoids mammograms, breast self-exam, the mention of the words "breast cancer," and, of course, all women who have either been diagnosed or treated for the disease for fear of catching "it." To say these people are neurotic is an under-statement.

How does this person react to stress?

Sometimes the person we reach out to is well meaning and wants to be helpful, but anxiety gets in the way. Instead of feeling comforted, we feel frazzled.

> VICKI turned to her favorite cousin, Wendy, who was pleased that Vicki chose to confide in her. She insisted on moving into Vicki's apartment to be with her through surgery and recovery. Vicki wasn't sure if this was such a good idea since Wendy's family nickname was "Nervous Nellie." But Wendy pooh-poohed her own anxiety and moved in.
>
> Within two days Wendy had lost her house keys, run a red light, and backed into a car while pulling out of a parking space. Although the calamities were minor, they were sufficient to make both women realize that the plan wasn't working. They agreed that a better arrangement was for Wendy to move back home and telephone once a day.

The point of this vignette is that a diagnosis of breast cancer puts a lot of stress on our loved ones, as well as ourselves. If we know their track record is iffy when it comes to handling a crisis or coping with stress, then it doesn't matter how much they love us and want to help, they will probably wind up being ineffectual. We won't get our needs met and will feel frustrated with ourselves, as well as with the other person. In the face of a crisis, we don't need additional calamity and hysteria. A calm, reassuring friend is what is needed.

But if we find that we have already reached out to a family member/friend who doesn't handle stress well, don't panic. What we need to do is set very clear limits and boundaries as to what this person may or may not do to be helpful.

For example, a phone call once a day may be ideal and allows us to control the length of the conversation. An actual visit is a bit trickier. It's hard to convince an anxious visitor that it's time to go home, without offending her generosity and causing even more stress.

Does this person know how to listen?

This may seem like a foolish question, but it isn't. Simply having ears on the side of your head is not enough. Listening is an art form which many claim to have mastered, but most need more lessons. Listening is not something you do while waiting for the other person to stop talking. Nor is it a contest in which you seize the first opportunity (usually a pause in mid-sentence) to jump in with a comment or switch to another subject.

A good listener is genuinely interested in what we have to say and the feeling behind the words. The responses are reflections of our words and feelings . . . or reactions to our actions. We set the tone and the mood. A good listener follows the lead, just like a good dance partner.

Interrupters and advice-givers are not good listeners. It's easy to spot them in conversation with others. They are the ones who talk too much and too often. When you are choosing people to reach out to for emotional support, select people who will encourage you to talk while they listen.

I know it may seem easier in the short run to let someone else do the talking while you do the listening, but I guarantee you will regret that choice in the long run. If you want to save yourself a lot of problems and depression *later*, find a good listener *now*.

When asked, is this person able to be objective and provide sound advice?

Sound advice consists of:

1. Encouraging you to communicate with your doctors when you have questions or want factual information. This includes asking the doctor for the names and phone numbers of knowledgeable patients who have been through this too, and are available to talk with you.

2. Suggesting that you weigh all the treatment options before making any final decisions. This may entail writing up a shopping list of advantages and disadvantages for each procedure you are considering, as well as seeking appropriate second opinions from qualified specialists.

3. Urging you to stay away from people who tell breast cancer "war stories," since they are exaggerations of the truth and only serve to scare you.

Bad advice from well-meaning people goes something like this:

1. "Why don't you try one of the laetrile clinics in Tijuana before you let them do surgery, chemotherapy, radiation, or all of the above?" (Suggestions that you try

unproven treatments *instead of* conventional methods are classic examples of bad advice.)

2. "It's all in your mind. If you think positive thoughts, you can cure the cancer yourself." (Positive thoughts *alone* do not cure cancer. You need medical treatment too.)

3. "Some breast cancers never get any larger and sometimes they even disappear. Why don't you wait six months to a year before you make any decisions?" (While it is true that some breast cancers can remain the same size for many years, no one can predict which ones will and which ones won't. In the meantime, the six months to one year that you wait may cost you your life.)

4. "Connie had breast cancer thirty years ago and she's still around today, so why don't you go for the same treatment she had?" (Connie had a Halsted radical mastectomy, an archaic disfiguring procedure that is rarely performed in this decade by state-of-the-art specialists.)

5. "Betty had very bad side effects from her treatment, so don't go for the same one she did." (Betty also gets carsick. Does that mean you're going to sell your car?)

Will this person maintain my confidences and refrain from discussing me with other friends and family members?

Let's face it, some people can't keep a secret, no matter what. Again, the best way to find out if the person is a blabbermouth is by looking at past performance. If this person calls you whenever she has a hot rumor about someone else, it's a cinch she will be calling someone else when she has a hot rumor about you.

Sometimes a friend or relative thinks she is being helpful and doesn't realize she is breaching a confidence.

DIANA discussed her diagnosis and treatment options with her daughter, Ellen. Ellen didn't think twice about talking to her aunt (Diana's sister) about her mother's condition, since her aunt had been treated for breast cancer a few years earlier and might have had some valuable information and family history to tell the physician that would affect treatment decisions.

It never dawned on Ellen that her mother didn't want her aunt to know what was going on until she was ready to tell her. Without meaning to cause trouble, Ellen stirred up a hornet's nest. The aunt was offended that Diana hadn't told her personally, Diana was hurt that her daughter had taken it upon herself to inform family members of the diagnosis without her permission, and Ellen was aggravated that no one appreciated her efforts.

How can we avoid this type of problem? When we confide in those close to us, it is extremely important to emphasize that:

1. We are going to take personal responsibility for telling friends and family members of our diagnosis, but not until we are ready and want them to know.

2. If anyone is in doubt as to who knows and who doesn't know, all they need to do is ask us.

3. We have our own reasons for keeping this information from certain people, and we expect our wishes to be respected.

4. If anyone feels that a particular person must be told immediately, they should explain why, and we will decide whether to disclose the information.

The incident with Diana's daughter and sister is just such a case in point. If Ellen had first explained to her mother why she felt her aunt should be told (rather than taking it upon herself to spill the beans), Diana might have agreed with Ellen's point of view and there would have been no hassle.

Some women have less need to keep this information a secret and decide to go public with it before the gossip-mongers do. They tell family members, friends, and neighbors of the diagnosis, not with the intention of receiving emotional support from everyone, but rather to get the facts straight before others have a chance to inadvertently distort them. Not a bad idea.

One of the secondary benefits of being open about your diagnosis and treatment is that you will receive unexpected emotional support from women you have met but never knew had breast cancer (neighbors, for instance). And if you are very public about it (that is, participate in breast cancer seminars or local newspaper, television, and radio interviews during the American Cancer Society's Breast Cancer Awareness Week), you will receive emotional support from breast cancer patients whom you have never even met or ever dreamed existed! And it wouldn't surprise me if some of those women became your close friends and support network.

For the record, I am not advocating going public, nor am I recommending remaining secretive. There are advantages and disadvantages to each, and once again it's a matter of preference—*your* preference, not your friends' or your family's.

This brings us to yet another thorny rose: peer support. When it's good, it's very, very good. And when it's bad, it's a disaster.

When is peer support helpful and when is it harmful?

Peer support can be helpful when:

1. We are going through treatment and recovery. It is beneficial to talk with other women who are going through the same experience and have similar concerns. We can swap anecdotes that make us laugh, others that make us cry, and in general have one hell of a catharsis letting it out!

2. We are newly diagnosed and our doctor gives us specific names and phone numbers of women who will provide us with accurate information and good emotional support.

Many of us assume that once a woman is treated for breast cancer she is an expert on the subject and will be helpful. This is not always true.

Peer support can be harmful when we are newly diagnosed and want other breast cancer patients to help decide what's best for us.

GRACE received her diagnosis on Monday. The next day she contacted a friend of a friend who was treated for breast cancer to advise her on treatment options. Instead of helping her to formulate a sensible plan and easing her anxiety, the woman got into a gripe session. She complained about long-term side effects, short-term side effects, problems with her doctors, family, employer, and friends. By the end of the conversation, Grace was feeling overwhelmed and scared. She got more than she bargained for, but none of it helpful.

She considered running away from treatment altogether, but thought better of it, and instead called her doctor. She told him how she felt, and he offered her a helpful solution. He put her in touch with two of his patients, each of whom had been treated with procedures that Grace was considering. These women were supportive and happy to answer her questions. There were some questions they couldn't answer, so they wisely referred her to the doctor. This time around she got what she needed and felt much less anxious.

There are two points to be made here. First, the type of peer discussion that is cathartic and meaningful when we are in treatment or going through recovery is too disruptive and disorganizing when we are trying to adjust to the diagnosis and make treatment choices. Second, peer support was never intended to help women make treatment choices. Here's why:

1. A woman who has elected mastectomy/reconstruction has no more knowledge about lumpectomy/radiation treatment than you do. In fact, you probably have the most current information since you were diagnosed more recently than she was. Obviously, the converse is also true. A woman who has chosen lumpectomy/radiation is not the best person to give expert advice on mastectomy/reconstruction.

2. Even if you are planning to have the same treatment as this woman, it may not be the identical procedure. For example, there are numerous types of reconstruction that follow mastectomy. With lumpectomy, there are two variations of radiation procedure. Similarly, there are several forms of chemotherapy.

3. Let's assume your treatment is the same and the procedure is identical. And you also have her team of doctors providing the care. It is still highly unlikely that your breast cancer is the exact size and type as hers. The size of your breast, as well as the size and type of the breast cancer, can greatly affect the cosmetic results and satisfaction with the outcome.

Someone who is pleased with her results is going to be more optimistic and upbeat than someone who is unhappy with the outcome. And just to complicate matters even further, since none of us are medical doctors specializing in breast cancer, we have no way of predicting whether our cosmetic results will be better, worse, or the same as someone else's who elected the same procedure.

4. Just because someone had breast cancer and has successfully recovered doesn't automatically make her interested in us or our breast cancer. Some women have absolutely no desire to network with other breast cancer patients, especially those who are newly diagnosed. It's too anxiety-provoking for them.

What is the best way to handle family members/friends who unintentionally upset you?

Try the direct approach. ("I really appreciate your concern, but let me call you when I'm not so anxious and more in the mood to talk.") If the direct approach gets you nowhere, go out and buy an answering machine to screen your calls. I'm serious about this. Where is it written that we have to pick up the phone and say hello just because it rings?

We can return calls when we're ready or not at all. We may recruit our spouse or some other family member to run interference for us and return phone calls to those we don't want to talk to.

Similarly, we can screen visitors too. Just because we are at home doesn't mean we must have company. If we don't want particular visitors, it's okay to tell them we aren't up to it and will contact them when we are. We may choose not to see or call them for several weeks or months. Believe me, we're not breaking their hearts. They are busy with their own problems and aren't waiting with bated breath to hear from us.

How do you know when friends and family aren't enough and you need to talk with a licensed psychotherapist?

It is time to look for professional help when:

1. We feel we are a burden on our loved ones. In some cases this is purely a figment of our imagination and doesn't reflect how our family and friends feel about us and our condition. In other instances, our perceptions are correct. Our loved ones feel emotionally drained and have no reserve energy left. They may become irritable or short-tempered, not because they are angry with us, but because they are exhausted and frustrated with the situation.

2. Our family members/friends don't seem to understand our feelings. It's hard for women who haven't had breast cancer to understand what this experience feels like. It may be even harder for men (for instance, your spouse or boyfriend) to recognize the emotional impact of this ordeal. Comments meant to be cheerful, such as: "Everything is going to be fine" or "It's only your breast, it's not your life," tend to convince us that our loved ones are not as empathic as we wish they were.

3. We don't want our family members/friends to know how we feel. There are two reasons for not wanting our loved ones to know how we feel:

   A. To protect ourselves from feeling even more misunderstood and/or burdensome to our family.

   B. To protect loved ones who we believe couldn't tolerate the shock, such as an elderly parent, a very young child, someone who is terminally ill or emotionally fragile.

4. We cast our family members/friends in the role of psychologist. This is a real set-up with a no-win outcome

for everyone. Even if our loved ones were professionally trained and licensed (which they probably aren't), they are too emotionally involved with us to be effective and constructive as our psychotherapist.

It's a mistake to look upon professional psychotherapy as the last resort to turn to after exhausting family and friends. The truth is that if psychotherapy were included in our treatment plan from the first day of our diagnosis, we wouldn't feel as if we were a drain on the people who love us. And there would be far fewer problems because we would have someone who, without becoming anxious or irritable, would keep our confidences safe and would help us control the unavoidable problems, while preventing or repairing the avoidable ones.

Professional support compliments personal support, and cuts through a lot of unnecessary tension for everyone. (See Chapter Five: Getting Professional Help: Sooner Is Better.)

The secret of success in reaching out to family and friends is: Be *realistic* about yourself and your loved ones. Recognize *needs* and *limitations*. Yours and theirs.

Summary

Family members/friends inadvertently fall into two camps:

> • Those who provide emotional support, love, and warmth.
> • Those who exacerbate our anxieties and fears.

We can learn how to maximize our interactions with the first group and minimize our interactions with the second group.

Points to consider before reaching out to a family member/friend include:

- What has my history been with this person?
- Are my expectations of the person realistic?
- Is this person "breast cancerphobic"?
- How does this person react to stress?
- Does this person encourage me to do the talking while he listens empathically without interrupting or giving advice?
- When asked, will this person provide objective, sound advice?
- Will this person maintain my confidences and refrain from discussing my problems with others?

Peer support from other breast cancer patients is usually helpful during treatment and recovery, but can be harmful immediately following the diagnosis.

We can learn how to handle family members and friends who unintentionally upset us and thereby avoid problems.

It's time to look for professional emotional support when:

- We feel we are a burden or drain on our loved ones.
- Our family and friends don't seem to understand our feelings.
- We don't want our loved ones to know how we feel.
- We cast our family or friends in the role of psychotherapist.

The secret of success in reaching out to family and friends is to be *realistic* about yourself and your loved ones and to recognize your *needs* and *limitations* as well as theirs.

CHAPTER FIVE

Getting
Professional Help:
Sooner Is Better

*T*he more I talk with patients, the more convinced I am that some type of professional psychotherapy needs to be included in our treatment plan. Preferably at the beginning. Why?

Many of us just don't get sufficient nurturing and healthy support from our family and friends. Even those of us who are fortunate enough to have solid, stable support systems find out fast there is a limit to how much we can tell our loved ones before they feel overwhelmed and we feel we are a burden to them.

Once we realize that friends and family are not enough, we are confronted with two choices:

1. Keep the excess feelings to ourselves and suffer in silence. This is clearly not our best choice since it leads to the classic avoidable problem of withdrawal and depression.

2. Find someone else to talk to who: a) understands the breast cancer experience without feeling intimidated by it; b) can help us sort out and express our feelings; c) will

help us cope more effectively when life feels like a three-ring circus without the laughs.

Enter the psychotherapist—ideally, one who specializes in working with cancer patients. If you don't know of such a person, your surgeon and oncologist will.

If psychotherapy is so helpful, why isn't it automatically included in our treatment plan?

Lack of awareness. Some doctors don't realize the extent to which breast cancer packs an emotional wallop. We add to this oversight when we pretend we're doing fine, even if we're really not.

Although most physicians acknowledge that breast cancer causes sadness and fear, many resist suggesting professional psychotherapy. Here are their reasons:

1. *"I can handle the patient's psychological needs myself."*
(Really? When was the last time your doctor sat down with you for forty-five to sixty minutes of uninterrupted conversation about your breast cancer and the feelings that accompany the diagnosis, treatment, and recovery?)

2. *"The patient might interpret it as an insult if I suggest that she needs psychotherapy."*
(Did you feel insulted when your doctor suggested you needed chemotherapy or radiation therapy? No. You probably felt scared, but knew it would help you, so you went for it. Psychotherapy is no different.)

3. *"Psychotherapy is too expensive and this patient is already concerned about the cost of her breast cancer treatment."*
(Your health insurance may cover some or all of the cost of your psychotherapy treatment. [See page 92.] And if it

doesn't, every community has free or low-fee psychotherapy available to those who qualify. If you are broke and
trying to cope with the emotional impact of breast cancer,
you qualify with a capital Q. Call your local American
Cancer Society, the Cancer Hotline [1-800-4-CANCER],
or the National Alliance of Breast Cancer Organizations
[1-212-719-0154] for help in locating an appropriate psychotherapist.)

4. *"If the patient is interested in psychotherapy, she already
has a therapist or knows of several to go to."*
(Not true. Most people don't get interested in psychotherapy until they have a problem. It's not a form of entertain-
ment or a hobby. You don't turn to your spouse and say
"Honey, what shall we do tonight? See a movie, go bowling,
or talk to a psychologist?")
  If you are presently in therapy with someone you like,
then by all means stick with it. If you have been in therapy
in the past and want to return to that person, do it now!
But if you don't have a therapist, past or present, this is
the time to ask your doctor for a referral.

Is there a best time to get into psychotherapy?

Yes. The best time is when we first get the diagnosis. But
the most popular time appears to be after we feel we have
exhausted our family and friends and have no one "safe"
to turn to.
  There are four critical stages in the breast cancer odyssey when anxiety, fear, and misinformation run rampant,
and psychotherapy can make the going a lot less rough.
They are:

1. Adjusting to the Diagnosis

2. Making Treatment Choices

3. Experiencing Side Effects of Treatment

4. Ending Treatment

During these four critical times, a competent psycho-therapist can help ease the confusion, stress, and feelings of helplessness and hopelessness. If the therapist has a special interest in breast cancer, she will be able to provide you with accurate breast cancer information, as well as refer you to current reading material. (See Appendix A: Suggested Reading List.)

1. *Diagnosis.* This is when your world falls apart and so do you. Although it's ideal to begin psychotherapy imme-diately after receiving the diagnosis, most of us are too stunned to think of it ourselves.

> ILENE: "I was like Humpty Dumpty after the fall. Splat! I'm lucky that my sister gave me the name of a good psycholo-gist and I went for help. The therapist picked up the shattered pieces of me. She became the glue that held me together so that I could get through treatment without cracking. When I was with my therapist, I could say what I was thinking and I didn't feel ashamed or alone. I could talk about my worst fears without upsetting my husband and kids."

2. *Choosing Treatment.* In a matter of days you are ex-pected to learn and understand a new language called "oncology" (that took your doctors years to learn) and become sufficiently expert to make treatment decisions that will affect the rest of your life.

JANET: "Everybody in the family was an expert when it came to choosing my treatment. Nobody was a doctor or ever had breast cancer, but they all thought they were experts. They drove me crazy. Not only did each one have a different idea of what I should do, but they kept changing their minds from day to day.

I finally decided, who needs this? I went to the psychologist my doctor recommended. Together, we weighed the emotional advantages and disadvantages of each possible treatment, until I reached my own decision. I thought I could do it in one visit, but it took more time. I didn't mind because it made a big difference in how I felt about myself, my family, and the breast cancer."

3. *Side Effects of Treatment.* It's spooky when you don't know what's going on with your body and can't figure out why you feel so lousy. You begin to ask yourself, "Is it the cancer, the treatment, my emotions, or some new illness unrelated to all of the above?"

KELLY: "I was depressed all of the time, had no appetite, and was losing weight. The doctor said it was from the chemotherapy treatment. I didn't believe him and told him that I knew what he really meant was that the chemo wasn't working and that my condition was getting worse. He sent me to a psychologist and she helped me get back the feeling of hope that I had lost along the way. I relaxed, gained weight, and got through the rest of the chemo with much less anxiety."

4. *End of Treatment.* It can be tough coming to grips with the reality that all of the army troops have gone home. There's only one lone soldier left on the battlefield—you!

LAUREL: "I had no problem that I couldn't handle until the week before my radiation treatment ended. And then I had a panic attack. I guess I was denying the whole breast cancer experience and it finally caught up with me. As much as I looked forward to the last day of radiation, I was petrified to be without daily treatment or the doctor's staff scurrying around. My husband couldn't understand it and neither could I. When I went into psychotherapy, I found out that I was afraid the cancer would return unless I saw my doctors every day. I began to realize how many thoughts and fears I had swept under the rug and hadn't looked at, beginning with the day I got diagnosed."

What are the various types of psychotherapy and how do you know which one is best for you?

There are three basic types of psychotherapy: individual, group, and family. And as you might have already guessed, there are pros and cons to each.

INDIVIDUAL PSYCHOTHERAPY: What's great about individual psychotherapy is that the focus is solely on you and your thoughts and feelings. You set the pace, and the therapist follows. You raise the issues when you are ready to deal with them and not before. If you have the financial means, it's the treatment of choice because it's tailored to your individual needs. This is particularly important during the four critical stages.

What's not so great about individual psychotherapy is the cost. It's expensive compared to group psychotherapy. Some of my patients who are on strict budgets have opted for individual psychotherapy on an as-needed basis with ongoing group psychotherapy on a regular weekly basis.

GROUP PSYCHOTHERAPY: Group therapy has two nifty things going for it. First, the price is right. Second, it's a good opportunity to make friends and share experiences with other women who have a wide range of thoughts and feelings about their own breast cancer experiences.

But all that glitters is not gold in group therapy. Many groups are limited to six to eight sessions. While some women find this adequate, others are just starting to blossom as the group ends and resent having to stop so soon.

On the other hand, some groups never even get anywhere. For example, sometimes there is a personality clash between members that doesn't get resolved and spoils the group atmosphere for everyone else.

MADELINE and NORA were just such a case in point. At the first meeting, each discovered she was treated by the same surgeon. Madeline had a positive experience, while Nora had a negative one. Every week they argued over the surgeon's competence and attempted to get the other group members to take sides. Despite the group leader's efforts, neither woman was willing to quit bickering or resign from the group. The animosity between them grew so thick that after one month, the group finally decided that the experience was so unpleasant and draining on everyone, that it would disband.

Another thought to take into consideration is whether your personality style lends itself to a group situation. It's not unusual for a couple of talkative women to take up a lot of the session time, leaving the quiet ones speechless (literally and figuratively). Even though the leader will make efforts to draw the quiet ones into the conversation, she won't do it forever, and, besides, it's really up to you to jump in without being coaxed. For this reason, group therapy works better for extroverts than introverts.

PAULA compared her group experience to watching a soap opera. She listened attentively to everyone, thinking to herself that her problems weren't nearly as bad as theirs. She never told anyone what was bothering her, even though the leader asked each week if there was anything she wanted to discuss. Once or twice she came close to speaking up, but changed her mind because her problems seemed too trivial compared to the others'.

After a month, the leader suggested that she might feel more like talking if she were in individual therapy. Paula realized this was true but was reluctant to give up the weekly camaraderie of the women. So she reached a compromise. She began individual therapy and met with the women in the group each week for coffee and friendship. Fortunately, both the therapy and the peer support flourished.

I find that groups can be very helpful once treatment has begun and especially during recovery. I am less enthusiastic about recommending group therapy when we are newly diagnosed and still weighing our treatment alternatives. Why?

A good, healthy group therapy situation is based on democratic principles. The majority rules. If the group's needs don't match your needs, you aren't going to get what you came for, and you may wind up feeling more confused when you leave than when you entered. Also, because time is of the essence, you need a lot of individualized attention, and the group can't give you this without neglecting other members.

An ideal situation is group therapy combined with individual treatment. Unfortunately, many of us don't have enough time or money to do both. If you are able to manage both, you won't regret your investment.

FAMILY THERAPY: Family psychotherapy includes couples therapy. Sometimes couples therapy is also known as conjoint therapy. No matter what you call it, the purpose is the same: to help you and your partner or other family members cope more effectively with your breast cancer. Sometimes your participation in the sessions will be required. At other times, you may be asked to stay away from the session. If this should happen, don't be alarmed. No one is conspiring against you. Frequently, psychotherapists find that family members are more apt to honestly disclose their feelings when the patient is not present.

> Roxy's husband, Jeff, felt he had to be strong for his wife and not let on that he was just as scared as she was. When I spoke to them together, he pretended he was fine. When I spoke to Jeff alone, he poured out his heart and revealed that he was worried sick.
>
> The goal of the treatment became clear—open and honest communication with one another, a sharing of their worst fears. A named fear is much less intimidating than one that you dare not speak.

Another example:

> SUZANNE never told her eleven-year-old daughter, Tina, that she was being treated for breast cancer. The child began having nightmares shortly after Suzanne's surgery but refused to tell her mother what the nightmares were about. When I talked to Tina alone, she revealed the secret. In the dream her mother was devoured by the shark from *Jaws*.
>
> The goal of the family therapy was to reassure Tina that her mother was not going to be eaten by the "cancer shark," and to create a closer bond between Suzanne and Tina through careful and honest communication, so that she would be less angry and fearful of losing her mother.

I encourage each of my breast cancer patients to include her partner and family in the psychotherapy whenever possible. I have found that most partners are more than willing to participate in the treatment. They look forward to future sessions and are grateful for the opportunity to be heard.

Nevertheless, most men tell me they are only doing this for their wives' or girlfriends' sakes and not for themselves. Although this is not true, they really believe it. And it's not worth making a big deal about. So what should you do? Nothing. If your guy needs to protect his machismo, let it be. Breast cancer poses a threat not just to your feelings of control, power, and sexuality, but to your partner's as well. If he's willing to come in for psychotherapy and talk about these feelings, what difference does it make who he thinks he's doing it for?

The only disadvantage to couples/family therapy is the cost. The fee is similar to individual treatment. Many of my patients find that it is a good supplement to individual treatment on an as-needed basis.

If I choose individual psychotherapy, how long will I have to be in treatment?

That depends on you, and what you want to accomplish. There are three traditional models of psychotherapy: crisis-oriented, short-term, and long-term.

Crisis-oriented

Treatment is brief, intensive, usually takes place within two weeks, and with a maximum of eight sessions. The purpose is to help you calm down, organize your thoughts, and formulate a clear and realistic plan. The trauma of adjusting to the diagnosis lends itself very well to crisis intervention . . . and so does the process of selecting a treatment plan, the team of doctors, and a hospital admission date.

Pro: It's economical in both time and money. A lot can be accomplished relatively quickly. It can keep you from falling apart. (If this has already occurred, it can quickly put you back together.) Assuming you have already acquired good coping skills elsewhere, and you have a healthy, reliable, personal support system, this may be the only psychotherapy you will need throughout your breast cancer experience.

Con: For most of us, it's like putting a Band-Aid on a gaping wound. There are so many issues and nuances to deal with from one day to the next that it's naive to believe you can cover all of them in half a dozen sessions. Because of the time limits, crisis intervention doesn't teach you coping skills for the future or how to problem solve. This means that if we haven't already acquired the knack of coping effectively, we are likely candidates for another crisis at the next critical stage.

Short-term

Treatment may vary from a few months to one year. The majority of my patients find that the full range of breast cancer issues can be adequately covered during twelve months since most of us are well into the recovery stage by the end of the first year.

Pro: If you stay in treatment for a year (without bringing in new problems), it's reasonable to expect to: increase your self-esteem; learn how to communicate more effectively with your family, friends, team of doctors,. and their staffs; come to terms with core issues such as fear of recurrence and death.

Con: Time and money. If you want to maximize your gains in short-term therapy, you will see your therapist no less than once and preferably several times a week. This can be expensive, as well as difficult to schedule, unless you and your therapist are willing to work evenings or weekends.

Long-term

This is the Rolls-Royce of psychotherapy. The question is, do you really need a Rolls-Royce? We are speaking of treatment lasting a minimum of one year and usually longer. There is no maximum number of years for treatment to last. In other words, the end of therapy is mutually determined by you and your therapist.

Some people in long-term psychotherapy see their therapists two to three times a week. This is in-depth treatment. In addition to addressing all of the short-term issues discussed above, you have the opportunity to resolve unfinished business from your past. I'm referring to old issues and conflicts that existed long before you were diagnosed with breast cancer.

For example, many of us experience our breast cancer treatment as an emotional turning point in our lives. It's as if it were a signal that it's time to make major changes in areas of our lives that are troublesome. For some of us it means making a career or life-style change. For others, it means straightening up or getting out of an unhappy relationship with a lover, husband, parent, or child. Or perhaps we simply want to come to terms with emotional wounds that date back to childhood and adolescence. Long-term psychotherapy gives you the time, space, and courage to come to grips with such matters.

Pro: It certainly rattles every skeleton out of the closet, examines each one with a fine-tooth comb, and then lays them to rest once and for all, so that we are no longer haunted by their presence. It also encourages us to make major changes in our lives that would have been difficult to achieve on our own.

Con: Not everyone has a skeleton in the closet. And even if we do, we may not want to rattle it, either now or later, let alone examine it in exquisite detail. And if we aren't interested in making major life-style changes and have no conflicts nipping at our heels from our early years, then long-term therapy is not a necessity, but rather a luxury, like a Rolls-Royce.

At one time or another, I have been a patient in each of the therapies I have described. I can't honestly say that one is better than the other. Much of it depends on you and what you want to get out of your treatment. What is most important for you to keep in mind is that each type of treatment has its limitations, and your expectations need to reflect that reality. For example, if you elect crisis intervention to hold you together while you adjust to the diagnosis, that's exactly what you can expect to get. Nothing more, nothing less. You will not learn coping skills to get you through the next potential crisis. For that, you will need short-term treatment, which is more costly and time-consuming. Ditto for long-term therapy, which can address more complicated issues and in greater detail than short-term treatment permits.

Does the sex of the therapist make a difference?

Only if it does to you. Theoretically, it makes no difference whether you are in treatment with a man or a woman, provided both are equally competent. Some of us have no particular preference, while others of us are absolute fanatics on the subject.

Personally, I was adamant about seeing a female therapist—not only a woman, but one who was treated for breast cancer too!

I wanted someone who had successfully recovered (physically and psychologically) so that she could serve as a light at the end of the tunnel. What I really needed was a role model. There are many of us who share these sentiments. On the other hand, there are many who don't.

Some women feel they relate better to men than to other women and, if given a choice, prefer their company. Since feeling comfortable with the psychotherapist is essential for successful treatment, it is foolish to agonize over the sex of the therapist. If you are more comfortable with a male therapist, go for it! There is nothing strange or unhealthy about your preference. Besides, if you are really curious as to why you prefer a male therapist instead of a female (or vice versa), you can always analyze the reasons at a later date with your therapist.

Are self-help groups a type of psychotherapy?

Technically speaking, the answer is no because there is no trained, licensed psychotherapist leading the group. Therefore we can't call it psychotherapy. But if you think about the spirit or purpose of psychotherapy, then the answer is yes, because anything that helps us to cope more effectively with breast cancer is, by definition, therapeutic.

I have participated in numerous breast cancer self-help groups, initially as a patient and later as a guest speaker. My experiences were very mixed, ranging from excellent to awful. Some groups were informative and friendly, and I looked forward to the next meeting, while others were hostile, depressing, and gave new meaning to the expression "Misery loves company, especially miserable company." I encourage participation in self-help groups that make you feel better for having been there. I discourage participation in self-help groups that leave you feeling down in the dumps or scared.

What are some red lights to watch for when you attend self-help groups?

- Gossiping about members who aren't present to defend themselves.

- Encouraging you to seek out specific physicians in the community (usually while trashing the reputations of others).

- Giving advice about treatment.

- Passing along "facts" when they are rumors and haven't been checked out.

- Feeling worse when you leave than when you arrived.

What are some green lights to look for when you attend self-help groups?

- Members encouraging each other to express their feelings without fear of being judged.

- A concerted effort on everyone's part to refrain from playing the role of psychotherapist and/or giving medical advice.

- Sharing recent newspaper and magazine articles about breast cancer that stimulate discussion in the group.

- Informing the group of upcoming events related to breast cancer (such as TV programs, films, lectures, conferences, etc.) that are of mutual interest.

- Inviting breast cancer specialists from your community to participate in informal rap sessions and answer questions.

- Feeling better for having attended and looking forward to the next meeting.

Using the above guidelines, you are now in a position to evaluate whether your self-help group is beneficial or detrimental to your emotional well-being.

Is psychotherapy covered by health insurance?

Health insurance companies insist that in the past, they have been taken to the cleaners paying off psychotherapy claims. Consequently, most health insurance carriers have made a substantial cut in mental health coverage. For example, some have a fixed dollar amount (i.e., $25 per session) regardless of how much your therapist charges (be it $25 or $125 per visit). Others have a fixed number of sessions per year (i.e., 20 visits), and still others have a maximum dollar amount per year (i.e., $1,000).

A good rule of thumb is to call your health insurance claims representative and find out what your *out-patient mental health benefits* are. Ask for specifics. For example, if you are told they will pay fifty percent of a reasonable and customary fee, ask them to tell you what the customary fee is in your particular community. Make sure you ask if there is a maximum number of sessions or dollar amount they will pay each year. Don't assume your coverage is based on the calendar year (January 1 to December 31). Many employers use a fiscal year (July 1 to June 30). Others use a benefit year that is determined by your first day of employment with the company. It is in your best interest to have all of this information at your fingertips when you discuss fees with your prospective psychotherapist. A growing number of psychotherapists, particularly those of us who work with cancer patients, use a sliding-scale fee based on ability to pay. When you know what your insurance will cover, it makes it a lot easier for you and the therapist to determine and agree on an affordable fee.

One final thought on this subject—bring your Description of Benefits booklet with you to your first session and ask your psychotherapist to double-check the coverage with either your claims representative or directly with the health insurance company. That way there will be no unpleasant financial surprises later on—for you or your therapist.

Summary

Some type of psychotherapy needs to be included in our treatment plan. The best time to begin is immediately following the diagnosis.

There are four critical stages in the breast cancer odyssey when psychotherapy can help alleviate a lot of our anxiety, fear, and misinformation. They are:

- adjusting to the diagnosis
- choosing treatment
- tolerating treatment side effects
- ending treatment

There are three types of psychotherapy: individual, family, and group. There are pros and cons to each. The one to choose is the one that feels the most comfortable.

How long we remain in psychotherapy depends on how much we want to accomplish. Crisis intervention is the quickest, but lacks depth. Long-term is the most thorough, but consumes a lot of time and money. Short-term is a compromise between the two. All three have merit.

Does the sex of the therapist make a difference? In theory, no. In practice, yes. If you have no preference, then it doesn't matter whether you go to a man or a woman. But if you have strong feelings one way or the other, then it will make a big difference. Follow your instincts.

Although self-help groups are not psychotherapy, they can play an important role in the breast cancer experience by providing friendship and information. Some of us seek out self-help groups instead of psychotherapy. A better idea: Try both.

Health insurance coverage for psychotherapy varies a great deal from one policy to another. Be an informed consumer and find out the details of your coverage *before* you meet with your therapist. That way, you can intelligently discuss an affordable fee. Bring the Description of Benefits booklet with you so that the psychotherapist can double-check the specifics of your coverage.

CHAPTER SIX

The Psychological

Effects of Our

Treatment Decisions:

Lumpectomy, Mastectomy,

Reconstruction

*D*o yourself a big favor. Before you make any final decisions about treatment, get a second opinion on your diagnosis. Have your biopsy slides read by another pathologist who is affiliated elsewhere. As unlikely as it is that the first pathologist misread the biopsy tissue, or that your slides got mixed up with someone else's, you owe it to yourself to make sure that no mistakes were made. The alternative is to worry and wonder for the rest of your life whether you were diagnosed accurately. And, in turn, whether you received correct treatment.

Does this seem far-fetched? It isn't. Our doctors base their treatment considerations and recommendations on the diagnostic information they receive from the pathologist. If the diagnosis is wrong or incomplete, it is logical that the rest of the procedures that follow will be too.

Neither the surgeon nor the oncologist makes the actual diagnosis. The pathologist does. The pathologist sends a written report of the findings to the doctor, who, in turn, passes on the information to us. Therefore, getting a second diagnostic opinion from another surgeon or oncologist is meaningless, since they will read the same piece of paper the first doctor did. What we really need is a second pathologist to examine the same biopsy slides from a fresh perspective and then give an opinion. Most of us aren't aware of this. You cannot assume that a second opinion on your treatment options will automatically include a diagnostic review of the biopsy slides, *unless you specifically request it.*

You may be asking yourself, why is she making such a big deal about the diagnosis? Here's why: Diagnosing breast cancer is not such a simple matter, especially with early breast cancer. That's when there is likely to be a complex range of diagnostic possibilities that some pathologists will call cancer requiring treatment and others will call a borderline condition that requires close observation, but no treatment.

If we are in that gray area, we should be apprised of it in order to make an informed decision regarding further surgery. We need to seriously consider the implications of additional treatment vs. no treatment. Therefore, we owe it to ourselves, for medical as well as psychological reasons, to get a second opinion from another pathologist.

Unless our health insurance coverage requires it, many of us never go for a second opinion. Here are some reasons:

1. *"I was afraid the doctor would be hurt or angry with me."*
That's the most popular one. What we need to realize is that competent physicians don't resent second opinions, and many welcome our desire to actively participate in the treatment. On the other hand, incompetent physicians are

threatened by second opinions, and well they should be! And well that we should be rid of them!

2. *"I didn't think it was necessary."*
Our doctors are not gods, even though a few of them would argue the point. Each of us wants to believe that our doctor is incapable of error. But given that they are human, they also have flaws, and the odds are they will goof up once in a while. Better it shouldn't be on us.

3. *"I didn't know I was supposed to."*
Now you do, and hopefully you will pass this information on to other women who need to know. This is a perfect example of not getting the kind of information/ advice we need when we are diagnosed. Whoever said "Ignorance is bliss" was definitely not a patient advocate.

4. *"I didn't want to spend the money."*
Nobody does. Don't despair. Most health insurance will pay for second opinions. Some even insist on it. Like you, they also have a vested interest in making sure the diagnosis is correct and the treatment is necessary. There's one big difference, however. Their motivation is purely financial.

Even if your health insurance doesn't cover the cost, do you really want to scrimp on your own life? Be a sport and spend the money. The price you pay in the short run will give you the tranquility you need in the long run.

When I was diagnosed with an early breast cancer, I didn't get a second opinion on my diagnosis or treatment options. Nobody suggested I should, and I didn't have the smarts to figure it out for myself. Granted, I was so swept away by the terror of having a life-threatening disease and my desperation to be rid of it that it never dawned on me that the diagnosis, as well as my treatment choice, deserved further scrutiny. I paid a price for that error.

Over the next year and a half, as my interest in and knowledge of breast cancer increased, so did my awareness of the controversial issues in the field. I discovered that early breast cancer diagnosis and treatment were subject to heated arguments among the specialists. Specifically, there was major disagreement over when to call it cancer and what treatment to recommend.

My anxiety level soared sky-high. Had I received an accurate diagnosis and subsequent treatment? Who knew? This was exacerbated further when, six months after treatment, I had a biopsy in my other breast and the findings were benign. Instead of being thrilled that I didn't have a second breast cancer, I became depressed and wondered if I really had had a first breast cancer six months earlier.

I spent many months agonizing over whether the diagnosis was correct. If it was, had lumpectomy/radiation been the right treatment choice? If the diagnosis was incorrect, had I jeopardized my future health by exposing my breast to high doses of radiation? Since it was all after the fact and neither the surgery nor the radiation could be undone, did I really want to pursue the truth? Was it better to let sleeping dogs lie? What if the doctors were wrong? Could I ever forgive them? What if the doctors were right? Could they ever forgive me for doubting them? And on and on and on, until I realized I was going to have insomnia for the rest of my life unless I got to the bottom of this . . . one way or another. So I got a belated but sorely needed second opinion.

With great trepidation, I had my biopsy slides and records sent to a well-respected breast cancer specialist. His pathologist carefully examined them. I purposely picked someone whom my doctors admired and felt a healthy rivalry toward. I figured the competition wouldn't hesitate to find fault.

Guess what? The diagnosis was correct. It was indeed a bona fide early breast cancer. And my treatment choice of lumpectomy/radiation? He concurred with that too.

Did I feel foolish? A little. But not enough to lose sleep, as I had for the previous year and a half. Did it create a problem in the relationship with my doctors? No. If anything, I may have gained their respect. One of them wondered why it took me so long to get around to checking! Would I do it again? Without a doubt. But this time I would do it *before* I made my treatment decision, instead of after.

So where do you go to find another pathologist? Better yet, since this can be a tricky judgment call, where do you find a pathologist who is an expert in breast cancer? Your surgeon and/or oncologist will know who the pathology specialists are, and will send your slides for review. Or, if you prefer, you can obtain your biopsy slides, consult with a second surgeon or oncologist, and have his/her pathologist give a second opinion. (Obviously, you need to make certain that the first and second pathologist aren't one and the same person.) Unless you live in a major city where there are pathologists who routinely diagnose breast cancer, your biopsy slides may have to be sent out of town for proper evaluation. It's worth the temporary inconvenience for the permanent peace of mind.

As soon as we are confident that the diagnosis is accurate, we are ready to move on to treatment decisions. This is the appropriate time to get second opinions from our general surgeon, reconstructive surgeon, oncologist and/ or radiation-oncologist.

Please keep in mind, however, that our doctor's area of expertise is likely to influence his recommendation. Specifically, radiation oncologists tend to favor lumpectomy/ radiation, while reconstructive surgeons tend to prefer mastectomy/reconstruction. It's not as self-serving as it first seems. I have found that most breast cancer specialists really do believe their specialty is the treatment of first choice—even when they aren't going to personally provide the treatment.

TRACY told the physicians with whom she consulted that she was planning to have her treatment in another city, so that she could recuperate at her sister's home. She wondered if knowing they wouldn't be providing the treatment would make a difference in their recommendations and attitude.

She talked with half a dozen specialists. All six doctors recommended the procedure they specialized in, even when they knew someone else would be performing the treatment. Three doctors made no attempt to convince her to stay. And of those three, one doctor referred her to several specialists in the other city. And that's the one she chose to remain with.

Most of us use majority rule when choosing surgical treatment. We tend to select the treatment that is recommended by the majority of doctors with whom we consult—be it one, two, or ten. Besides the pathologist's report, which gives the size and type of the breast cancer, do our doctors use any other information to determine treatment recommendations? Yes. The other factors are: the size of the lump in ratio to the size of our breast, our age, our physical health, our family history of breast cancer (family history is a controversial issue; many specialists believe a positive history for breast cancer should not discourage you from choosing lumpectomy/radiation, if you so desire), and, last but not least, those treatment procedures that have succeeded in the past. The psychological factor is often dismissed or forgotten.

We are the ones who must live with the results of our treatment decisions, for better or worse. For that reason, it's hard to believe that we would purposely avoid finding out about potential psychological effects, if only the information were offered to us. I cannot emphasize enough the importance of taking enough time to weigh the psychological pros and cons of the various surgical procedures *before* making a final decision.

This leads us into an area of psychological resistance to

breast cancer treatment that I call "Don't mess with success." Sometimes well-intentioned people get stuck on what has worked in the past, refusing to consider any new and/or improved methods. For example, we all know that setting our hair with bobby pins works, but we now have more modern techniques for curling our hair that are at least as effective, and perhaps with more aesthetically pleasing results. So it is with breast cancer surgery. Here's a short history lesson that says it all:

There used to be a time when breast reconstruction following mastectomy wasn't even a remote possibility. It was considered medically unsound, as well as pandering to female vanity.

Eventually, those archaic notions were replaced with the belief that it was probably okay to do reconstruction, but only if the patient specifically requested it. And then we were required to prove our sincerity by waiting a few years because it was feared that if it were done sooner, we wouldn't fully appreciate our new breast.

With the passage of time, those ideas and attitudes were abandoned because scientific research demonstrated that the sooner we were reconstructed, the sooner we felt better about ourselves.

Current psychological thinking favors the idea of reconstructing as soon as it is medically safe. In some instances, it is feasible to do reconstruction at the same time the mastectomy is performed. If we opt for immediate reconstruction, it is a wise idea to arrange ahead of time to donate our own blood, should extra blood be needed during the surgery. Additional state-of-the-art thinking includes: a) automatically offering reconstruction as a treatment option rather than waiting for the patient to ask; b) making the mastectomy incision in a way that facilitates reconstruction should we decide we want it at a later date.

That's quite an evolution in attitude and thinking. Breast reconstruction in the United States has gone from medical scorn to medical acceptance, even praise, in a span of twenty-five years—thanks to the efforts of those women who made their feelings about reconstruction known. And thanks to those doctors who were open to new ideas and willing to listen and learn.

But that's not the end of the story by a long shot. No sooner did we slay one mythical dragon than another appeared on the horizon. And don't you know, it's still breathing fire. I'm talking about the lumpectomy/radiation treatment alternative.

Lumpectomy/radiation is the new kid on the block. And along with every newcomer to the neighborhood, there's always the gang of bullies who need to protect their turf. So they identify the newcomer as the enemy and this entitles them to beat up on him, hoping he will go back to where he came from (in this case, France, where lumpectomy/radiation has enjoyed success for more than twenty years). In the opposite camp, and equally as childish, is the adoring fan club. They have fallen head over heels in love with the new kid, insisting he will solve everyone's problems and will be all things to all people. The truth is the new kid is neither adversary nor salvation. If you doubt it, please remember there once was a time when breast reconstruction was the new kid on the block.

With the passage of time, we have come to recognize the virtues and shortcomings of breast reconstruction, medically and psychologically. And the same is true for lumpectomy/radiation.

What are the psychological advantages and disadvantages of the lumpectomy/radiation procedure?

Advantages:

1. Clearly, the greatest benefit is that we get to save our breast. This engenders a big sigh of relief in many of us.

It makes the threat of breast cancer far less frightening. After all, one of the main reasons women have avoided breast cancer screenings in the past is because we were afraid of losing our breasts if cancer were detected.

2. When we get good cosmetic results, no one but our doctors and ourselves is able to tell that we were treated for cancer, unless we choose to reveal it. This gives us more control over our lives and makes us less emotionally vulnerable to the unintentional insensitivity of others. This is an important factor for all of us, but especially for divorced and single women who may not wish to share their diagnosis and treatment with their prospective partners until a later time.

VANESSA found that when she told her new boyfriend she had been treated for breast cancer, he got nervous, seemed to distance himself from her, and ultimately it became impossible to establish intimacy between them.

When the relationship ended she decided to take a different approach with her next boyfriend. This time she waited until they knew each other for six months and the intimacy was established, both intellectually and sexually, before she told him of her treatment. It worked. He wasn't scared off. They grew closer together instead of further apart.

The favorable cosmetic result of her lumpectomy/radiation procedure gave Vanessa the option of disclosing her breast cancer treatment when she was ready to do so and not because her boyfriend was going to notice it first. (See Chapter Nine: Love, Sex, Dating and Marriage.)

3. It's one less stress to deal with. We can focus our attention and feelings on coping with the diagnosis, treat-

ment, and recovery, without having to contend with breast loss.

> ABBY was overwhelmed by the diagnosis. She was the only one in her family and the first of her friends to be treated for breast cancer. She had no one to compare notes with. Looking back on the experience, she felt that emotionally she was hanging on by her fingernails. "If there had been one more trauma to cope with, such as amputation of my breast, I would have gone over the edge."

I don't know that she really would have gone over the edge. But what is important is that *she* believed it. And it is *our* personal experience, not our therapist's opinion of that experience, that is most valid in helping us to understand, cope, and recover from the breast cancer trauma.

Disadvantages:

1. The *thought* of radiation scares the wits out of most of us. The *actual act* of having your breast irradiated scares the wits out of the rest of us. To put it simply, radiation is intimidating, both in thought and deed. And with good reason. For as long as we can remember, we have been told that radiation is dangerous and to stay away from it. Suddenly we are asked to take it on faith that for breast cancer, radiation is safe. It makes you wonder who and what to believe.

If you have a radiation phobia, this is not the treatment for you. You would spend the rest of your life looking for maladies and symptoms of radiation-induced illness, blaming every sniffle and sneeze on the treatment. Worst of all, you would anticipate developing another cancer caused by the radiation. Even those of us who aren't fearful of radiation occasionally wonder what the long-term effects of the treatment will be. A case in point:

BEVERLY developed numbness in her right leg approximately two years after her radiation treatment was completed. The neurologist couldn't find the cause, but recognized a mild and nonprogressive spinal cord injury. When she told him that she had had radiation to her breast, he told her the spinal cord injury was a side effect of the radiation.

Extremely upset, Beverly called the radiation oncologist and told him the news. The doctor calmly and correctly pointed out that her spine was nowhere in the radiation field and received no treatment. She realized this was true. The cause of the numbness was due to reasons unrelated to radiation treatment.

Even though we try hard not to become victims of radiation hysteria, occasionally we may fall into the trap, especially when provoked by physicians who are opposed to or are ignorant about radiation treatment for breast cancer.

2. When the cancer is large, a greater area of the breast tissue must be removed, and the cosmetic results are compromised and often less than pleasing. This can be very traumatic for someone who specifically chose this treatment because she wanted to keep her breast intact.

Why do women with large cancers choose this procedure in the first place? Although many of us feel there is no advantage in saving a distorted breast when there are excellent reconstructive procedures available, some of us feel it is important to preserve our own natural breast no matter what. Since there is no danger physically or psychologically, who's to say nay? After all, beauty is in the eye of the beholder.

3. When the radiation oncologist (also called the radiation therapist) isn't top-notch, two serious problems may occur: First, the aesthetic results can be unattractive, leaving us with feelings of disappointment and anger; a con-

viction that radiation doesn't work; and the belief that our doctors didn't know what they were doing. Second, if the breast, chest, and axillary node area aren't measured precisely, the radiation may not get to all of the fields that need to be treated, making a recurrence of the very same breast cancer a distinct possibility. Needless to say, this is a trauma that you don't want to repeat. Therefore, if you can't get to someone who specializes in breast radiation, don't elect this procedure.

4. If we are dissatisfied with the cosmetic results following lumpectomy/radiation treatment, further surgery (that is, mastectomy and reconstruction) may be awkward and delicate, although not impossible. Irradiated skin is difficult to work with and most surgeons would rather not. In other words, the bottom line is that it isn't so easy to change or convert a lumpectomy/radiation procedure into a mastectomy/reconstruction procedure. So be certain before you make the final choice.

5. Some of us elect lumpectomy/radiation and then get cold feet. After the lumpectomy, we change our minds about radiation and decide not to do it. This is like having the dentist clean out a cavity and then deciding not to put in the filling. It's a halfway measure at best that leaves you in medical jeopardy and therefore with eternal anxiety.

Unless your doctor tells you that for your type of early breast cancer radiation therapy is not mandatory, it is expected that you will complete the procedure with radiation treatment. This isn't a buffet where you take the best and leave the rest. It's a fixed menu. All or nothing. If you object to radiation, don't choose a lumpectomy. And above all, know what you are getting yourself into, or you are likely to find yourself up to your elbows in alligators.

What are the psychological advantages and disadvantages of mastectomy?

Advantages:

1. A simple surgical procedure removes the cancerous tissue. There is no worry about radiation-related illness, real or imagined.

> CEILE had an early breast cancer and was a good candidate for lumpectomy/radiation, except for one major factor. Radiation terrified her. She shuddered as she contemplated what the long-term effects of the treatment might be. Her husband felt the same way. They both agreed that mastectomy was preferable to living with radiation anxiety. For herself, Ceile made the wisest decision.

2. There is a longer proven track record for mastectomy than for lumpectomy/radiation, and there always will be. (Just as your older sister will always be your older sister, even when you are eighty-five and she is ninety.) If there is safety in numbers, it is comforting to know that, so far, the numbers of successful mastectomies outdistance the numbers of successful lumpectomy/radiation procedures. (Some say this is a weak argument and that what is important over the long term is the percentage of successes of each treatment.)

Disadvantages:

1. It's a double whammy, trying to adjust to losing your breast while simultaneously trying to cope with surviving a life-threatening illness.

2. If we have unresolved conflicts about our femininity, sexuality, or desirability, they are likely to surface as a result of the mastectomy.

> DORIS was single, introverted, and rarely dated. She never really felt attractive and was constantly dieting and working out at the gym to improve her appearance. The mastectomy was the final blow to her self-esteem and her hope of becoming a desirable woman in men's eyes. She felt ugly and hopeless about herself. She believed that not only would no man ever find her pretty and sexy, but now everyone would find her a pitiful creature. She quit her job and began to withdraw from all social activities. Fortunately, she entered psychotherapy before she became a total recluse. She now feels much better about herself and is dating more frequently than she did presurgery.

What are the psychological considerations in choosing breast reconstruction?

Breast reconstruction is an elective procedure. Although it is not a requirement for successful treatment of breast cancer, wanting reconstruction is a healthy emotional response, even if our *only* reason is to get rid of the physical feeling of lopsidedness and pronounced weight difference. But not every woman wants to have her breast reconstructed. Nor is it fair to say that if a woman decides against reconstruction, there is something psychologically wrong with her. Some women don't want any more surgery or pain, and they do fine with a breast prosthesis.

> EDIE was attractive, confident, successful, and happily married with several grown children. She had undergone numerous major surgeries over the previous ten years and the thought of more surgery, especially elective, was totally unappealing. Her husband concurred with her decision.

Neither one has regretted it. And if they ever do, she will have reconstruction.

There are other healthy reasons women decide against breast reconstruction. Women with strong feminist attitudes frequently decide not to reconstruct. They feel that femininity cannot be defined by two mounds of flesh. I believe the sentiment is valid, but it's not the best choice for everyone.

Not every reason for deciding against breast reconstruction is healthy. Some reasons are just excuses and rationalizations that indicate unresolved conflicts relating to self-worth and self-esteem:

1. *"My prognosis is poor. I'm going to die of breast cancer anyway, so why try and put up a good front? No pun intended."*
(At least this woman has a sense of humor. Nobody has a crystal ball that says how long we have on this earth. Yes, some of us do have a better prognosis than others. But so what? If you want to reconstruct, do it. Your pal with the great prognosis, who got reconstructed without giving it a second thought, may die by slipping on a bar of soap in the bathtub next month. And you with the not-so-hot prognosis, who chose not to reconstruct, may live for the next twenty-five years or longer. Do it with style and grace.)

2. *"When it comes to dating, I have no interest. So why bother?"*
(*You* are worth the bother, not the people you date. Do it for yourself or don't do it at all. If it will make you feel better about yourself, that's reason enough.)

3. *"I'm too old for that."*
(This was from a woman in her forties. So I asked, "At what age are we too old to have two breasts?" I recently treated a woman in her late seventies who had abdominal

flap reconstruction, which is the most difficult and complicated type. She didn't think *she* was too old. And neither
do I.)

4. *"It will never be the same as the natural one."*
(That's right. And it's also true that we will never be
twenty-one again or look as good in a bikini as we looked
then. So should we give up trying to look attractive because
we can't look sensational?)

5. *"I'm too depressed to even consider it."*
(Understandable. One way to pull yourself out of the
depression is to start making plans to do things that will
make you feel better about yourself. Reconstruction can
be a positive step in that direction. It's sure worth the
investigation. And the energy you spend gathering the
information may be the catalyst that lifts the depression.)

Is one type of breast reconstruction psychologically healthier than another?

No. The best one is the one that you find most appealing
and the surgeon feels will work best for you. Time and
money also need to be figured into your decision, as some
procedures are more costly than others, and some require
more weeks of at-home recuperation.

Here are some tips to make your decision less emotionally trying:

1. Have the reconstructive surgeon list the medical and
cosmetic pros and cons of the various procedures. Be sure
to have him/her include potential complications and side
effects.

2. Look at photographs of good and bad cosmetic results. I don't mean in magazines and textbooks. I'm talking about your doctor's photo album of his breast reconstruction successes and failures.

3. Ask the doctor how many breast reconstructions he has performed in the last year. The answer you get will tell you whether breast reconstruction is one of his specialties.

4. Some types of breast reconstruction are more difficult than others and require years of mastery. Find out from the doctor the number of breast reconstructions *of the type you are considering* he has performed. If the number is low, you may want to look elsewhere.

5. Ask the doctor to arrange a meeting with a couple of patients who were successfully treated with the type of reconstruction you are considering. There's nothing that will help you make up your mind faster than a good "look and feel."

Reaching the Final Decision

For many of us, the finality of arriving at the treatment decision is more anxiety-provoking than actually receiving the diagnosis. So many agonizing questions appear and reappear, begging for answers. For example: How much time do I have between diagnosis and surgery? How long is too long to wait? How do I know if I'm making the right decision? The factual answers to these questions are unknowable. It's a matter of opinion and personal choice. The decision you reach will be made easier if you follow this suggestion list.

The Don't *list includes:*

1. Don't listen to breast cancer treatment gossip from well-meaning friends and relatives. Most of it will be inaccurate or exaggerated.

2. Don't run away from making a decision. Yes, it's overwhelming and excruciatingly stressful, and you have every right to want to run. But don't do it.

3. Don't make an on-the-spot decision. You have more time than you realize. Experts say at least two weeks and up to one month.

4. Don't ask your partner to make the decision for you. You will always resent him for it.

5. Don't ask your friends and family what they would do. They aren't you. They don't have to live inside your body or your head.

6. Don't ask your doctor, "If I were your wife what treatment would you want me to have?" This is a temptation many of us succumb to (including yours truly). It seems like a dandy question to raise until you realize that you have absolutely no idea what his feelings are toward his wife. Does he have a warm loving relationship, or is he in the midst of a bitter divorce? Even more to the point is this: a recommendation that may be right for her emotional make up, may be wrong for yours.

The Do *list includes:*

1. Do read! Read! Read! Your doctors will know which books and magazine articles on breast cancer are current

and accurate. If they don't, then you're not with breast cancer specialists. If you read, you will gain a better understanding of the issues and choices, which in turn will lead to greater self-confidence that you are arriving at an informed decision. Knowledge is a powerful tool.

2. Do talk! Talk! Talk! Talk *to your doctors* to make sure you fully understand what was said. As mentioned in Chapter Two ("The Patient-Doctor Relationship"), this is when the cassette tape comes in handy. Replay it as often as you like. Some of us find the sound of our doctor's voice reassuring and soothing. Talk *to your psychotherapist* about your feelings and fears. Talk *to other patients treated by your physicians,* especially those who elected the surgical procedures you are contemplating. These women will be helpful and provide good emotional support as well. Talk *to family and friends,* but only those who will alleviate—not generate—anxiety. (See Chapter Four, "Choosing Personal Support Systems.")

3. Do take as much time as you need to make an intelligent and informed decision. Since there are no guarantees on longevity, the choice may as well be the one that you can best come to terms with.

4. Do keep in mind there is no one "right" treatment that works for everyone. What is right for your friend may not be right for you—medically, psychologically, and/or both.

5. Do sleep on your final decision for a night or two. Just to be sure!

Summary

Your treatment is only as accurate as your diagnosis. Before deciding on a treatment plan, run a double check on the biopsy slides to make sure the diagnosis is correct.

Take (or send) your biopsy slides to a pathologist who is affiliated elsewhere for a second opinion on the diagnosis. See another surgeon or oncologist for a second opinion on the treatment plan.

The reasons we don't go for second opinions include:

- We are afraid the doctor will be hurt/angry.
- We didn't think it was necessary.
- We didn't know we were supposed to.
- We didn't want to spend the money.

When discussing treatment options, keep in mind that each doctor may have an unintentional bias toward his/her medical specialty. That's why it's so important that the final decision be your own.

Factors to consider in choosing a treatment plan:

- type of breast cancer
- size of breast cancer
- size of breast in relation to size of breast cancer
- family history of breast cancer (debatable according to the experts)
- age
- physical health
- personal preference

The psychological advantages of lumpectomy/radiation:

- You get to save your breast.
- No one can tell unless you tell them first or they know what to look for.
- Less trauma than mastectomy because there is no breast loss.

The psychological disadvantages of lumpectomy/radiation:

- Like the high school tramp, radiation has a reputation that's hard to live down, much less forget.
- Fear of radiation-induced illness in the future stirs up a lot of anxiety and fear in the present.
- The skill of the radiation oncologist (also called radiation therapist) and the team of technicians can make or break the medical as well as the cosmetic results.
- If you don't like the cosmetic result, you may be stuck. It's difficult to do breast reconstruction on irradiated skin.

The psychological advantages of mastectomy:

- It's a tried and true method with a longer track record of success than lumpectomy/radiation.
- One procedure removes the cancerous tissue. There is no worry over radiation-related illness.

The psychological disadvantages of mastectomy:

- You have to adjust to breast loss at the same time you are coping with surviving a life-threatening illness.
- It can stir up unresolved conflicts about your femininity, sexuality, and desirability.

Not every woman wants breast reconstruction. But every woman who does should have it as soon as it is medically safe.

There are psychologically healthy reasons for not wanting breast reconstruction:

- Feeling attractive, confident, and successful without breast reconstruction.
- As a feminist statement against sexist values.

And there are psychologically unhealthy reasons for not wanting breast reconstruction:

- I'm going to die anyway.
- I'm not dating, so I don't need breasts.
- I'm too old to bother.
- It won't look as good as the original.
- I'm too depressed to consider more surgery.

There are several types of breast reconstruction. The best one is the one that most appeals to you and your doctor feels will give you good cosmetic results.

The quickest way to zero in on the type of breast reconstruction you want:

- Ask the doctor to list all medical and cosmetic pros and cons of each type, including potential complications and side effects.
- Check the doctor's breast reconstruction photo album. Ask to see the failures as well as the successes.
- Experience is highly desirable. Ask how many breast reconstructions of the type you want he performed in the last year.
- Have the doctor arrange a meeting with a couple of patients who have the type of reconstruction you want. They will "show and tell" and you will "look and feel."

CHAPTER SEVEN

The Low Down,
No Good,
Chemotherapy/Radiation
Blues

*I*f the cancer doesn't kill me, the cure will. The irony of the joke is clear to anyone who undergoes chemotherapy or radiation. Both have uncomfortable physical and psychological side effects that feel lethal. Most of the discomfort is short term, but there are long-term issues as well. Some of the difficulties are universal and unavoidable, while others are unnecessary and avoidable for those of us who are willing to get involved in our treatment.

We all need to vent our feelings about treatment side effects. It's irrelevant whether our symptoms are better/worse than someone else's. Besides, the very same side effect can feel mild to one person and severe to another. For example, one women in chemotherapy loses her hair and it's a nuisance, while another woman experiences it as trauma. Is one right and the other wrong? Absolutely not. Both are equally valid.

Another important piece of information to keep in

mind is the list of prizes awarded to those of us who stifle our feelings: depression, ulcers, alcoholism, and drug addiction, to name a few. Silence and stoicism are not signs of strength. They are signs of isolation and alienation. It's the last thing we need at a time like this.

If we are going to receive chemotherapy or radiation, it will most likely begin *after* some or all of our surgery is completed. Emotionally, this may feel like adding insult to injury. And it is! Barely adjusted to the physical and psychological trauma of the surgery, we must face yet another hurdle.

While there are vast differences between chemotherapy and radiation, many of the emotional side effects are similar. Let's look at the psychological issues these treatments have in common.

Universal/unavoidable questions and issues

1. *Are you sure this won't do me more harm than good?* If we haven't already posed this question to our doctor when chemotherapy or radiation was initially suggested, it is certain that the thought will occur to us just as soon as we experience our first unpleasant physical side effect. It's natural to wonder whether something that often makes us feel so bad can really be doing us any good.

Let's face it, when an intelligent woman subjects her body to toxic chemicals and/or massive doses of X-ray, it's reasonable to expect serious concerns about the short- and long-term effects. That's why it's so important for each of us to select breast cancer specialists whose medical expertise is worthy of our trust and who will take whatever time is necessary to talk with us, answer questions, and allay our fears. When in the hands of competent physicians, chemotherapy and radiation are never administered capriciously. They are prescribed only when there is reason to believe they will increase the duration and quality of life.

2. Is this ever going to end? (Or do I have to die first?) This complaint surfaces well into the treatment cycle, when our curiosity/fascination with our symptoms has worn off and we just want OUT. Enter the feelings of physical and emotional exhaustion. Mercifully, this is a temporary condition that disappears when we are through with treatment. Fatigue, however, can take up to a year to dissipate. So don't panic if you don't bounce back to your old self in a matter of weeks.

Not all of us receive an exact end-of-treatment date. Some of us may require additional chemotherapy or radiation after the initial therapy is evaluated. When this happens, it's understandably upsetting. It's a lot easier to hang in there when we can actually see the light at the end of the tunnel instead of having to take someone else's word for it. One way to make it *easier* (I'd be a fool to say *easy*) is to have nurturing support systems available.

Most of us receive *either* chemotherapy *or* radiation. But some of us lucky devils get to have *both*. It takes a lot of physical and emotional stamina to endure both therapies, one right after the other. It's not unusual for the total treatment procedure to last a full year. That's an incredibly long time to have your body invaded by foreign substances while simultaneously trying to keep your mental health from fraying around the edges.

Now please don't jump to the conclusion that I'm trying to minimize your five to six weeks of radiation or someone else's six months of chemotherapy, but just imagine what it would be like to endure both for an entire year, on top of the original breast surgery! And that's not including reconstruction!

One way to make the process emotionally bearable is to be good to ourselves. This requires special treats on a regular basis. For some of us it means buying frivolous items such as record albums, costume jewelry, and trinkets; or taking long weekends at our favorite seaside, mountain, or country inn; or going to the most elegant restaurant and ordering anything we darn well please without first checking calories or price.

> During the course of her radiation, FAYE fancied herself the queen of England (or at least Princess Di). Every Friday, dressed in her best designer outfit, she invited a girlfriend to join her for an outrageously snooty and aristocratic high tea that was also sinfully delicious and decadent. Oh sure, it was expensive for what it was (your basic pot of hot water and plate of cookies), but when compared to buying a pair of shoes or dress each week, a twelve-dollar tea bag was a real bargain.
>
> Adding to the pleasure was the fact that even though the scones, jam, cream, and pastries were very fattening, for the first time in her life she didn't have to worry about weight gain because the radiation curbed her appetite for all but easy-to-swallow foods. Needless to say, when the radiation ended, her appetite and weight returned to normal and she bid farewell to the highly caloric high teas.

If you're watching your weight, why not feast your eyes and ears instead of your stomach? Try theatre, films, concerts, art museums, and galleries. Many are free! If you're short on cash, try soaking in a long, luxurious bubble bath each night, or going to the local public library and checking out the books on the best-seller list that you've been meaning to read for the last year but never got around to. TV is always a good old standby, but please don't become a couch potato.

Whatever special treat you decide on, schedule it *frequently* and at *regular intervals*. For those of us in radiation, it means on the two to three nontreatment days each week. For those of us in chemotherapy, it means on our first "good" day following *each* treatment.

Psychologists have long understood the powerful effect

of pairing a pleasant event/activity *immediately following* an unpleasant one. The idea is to associate a positive experience (a romantic walk on the beach) following a negative one (the nausea that often accompanies chemotherapy treatment) and reward yourself (by taking the romantic walk just as soon as the nausea subsides). When we give ourselves something pleasurable to look forward to, the discomfort of the treatment side effects becomes more bearable. Of course there are subtle nuances that can help make this plan more effective. For example, a trip to Tahiti is not a good short-term reward because you can't go there until the entire treatment is completed. But tickets to the Wednesday night ballet might just hit the spot, and certainly won't interfere with your treatment. You may want to get some professional consultation to help you map out a workable reward system for yourself.

3. Fear of the unknown. This is a universal and unavoidable problem that is unique to life and not just to chemotherapy and radiation. The first treatment, like the first day of school, is always the scariest because we don't know what to expect. Will it hurt? Will I be able to handle it? What if I make a scene or decide to quit? And then suddenly our first treatment is over and we realize it wasn't as bad as we imagined, and that we can and will handle it.

It's a funny thing about fear of the unknown—even though it's a universal feeling, much of it can be circumvented if only we read the doctor's handout, especially *before* we arrive for our first session. Our doctors give us pamphlets explaining the whys and wherefores of chemotherapy and radiation, including what to expect before, during, and after treatment. Many of us neglect this preparation for a variety of reasons:

  A. In our anxiety, we forget that we were given the material or we misplace it.

B. We're afraid to read the pamphlet because it might increase our anxiety and scare us away from treatment.

C. We believe the situation is hopeless, so what difference would it make to read a brochure.

D. It's easier to listen to someone else's experience, however distorted it may be, than it is to read factual information.

E. We're still in a state of denial, believing this is a bad dream. Well, dear heart, it ain't a bad dream . . . it's a bad reality. And we have the power to make it better or worse.

If we don't read the pamphlets and absorb the information, we are setting the stage for avoidable problems. Granted, reading will not alleviate *all* of the fear of the unknown. But it will certainly cut through a lot of the nonsensical panic.

In her anxiety, GINA raced past the paragraph that said the radiation machine would make a loud buzzing noise. She was verbally reminded of this on the day she appeared for her first treatment. But she was nervous and didn't hear what was said. A few minutes later the machine was turned on. As predicted, it made a loud buzzing noise. Gina shrieked at the top of her lungs and screamed for help. She thought the machine was broken and that radiation was pouring all over her body. It took a while to calm her down and reassure her that everything was under control and there was no need to panic. She was embarrassed and later went home and read the pamphlet from cover to cover.

What's the lesson to be learned? Some of our fears of the unknown are, in fact, knowable and therefore avoidable, if only we are willing to take the time to acquaint ourselves with the nature of our treatment and listen to explanations from our doctors and their staffs. If we know that our anxiety prevents us from listening with a clear head, we can always bring in a family member, friend, or tape recorder for backup.

4. *Feeling fatigued and depressed.* Ever hear the expression, "I've been down so long, it looks like up to me"? That's what extended treatment for breast cancer feels like. You forget what it's like to be treatment-free. A certain amount of fatigue and depression is par for the course and unavoidable, due to the fact that radiation, and especially chemotherapy, use up a lot of our energy and this causes weariness. When we are tired, we become irritable and depressed. This is a simplistic but practical explanation, and essentially all we need to know in order to map out a plan to minimize our own exhaustion and depression. Here are some suggestions that can provide psychological comfort:

A. *Make eating easy.* If you like it, eat it. To combat weight loss and subsequent lack of energy, eat foods that you enjoy, and if they are not particularly nutritious, ask your doctor to give you vitamin supplements. Combating weight gain is a bit trickier, but not impossible. A balanced diet is always the ideal. However, some foods reduce nausea better than others, and these usually aren't the foods that are dietetic. Frankly, I feel that the worst time to go on a weight-reduction diet is while undergoing chemotherapy/radiation. It's too depriving, especially since we need to pamper ourselves during this period. There is plenty of time to diet when we are treatment-free and have less stress to contend with. Also, eating *more* rather than *less* is a basic survival instinct, dating back to early infancy. Babies who thrive are the ones who eat, and babies who succumb are the ones who don't.

B. *Stop fighting fatigue.* It's our body's way of asking for a mini-vacation called sleep. Respect the request. Take a nap. If this is out of the question, talk yourself into going to bed a couple of hours earlier each night, or if you prefer, sleep two hours later in the morning. Whatever the choice, plan for some extra sleep on a daily basis until the treatment is over. Remember, fatigue causes depression, irritability, confusion, and poor judgment. You're in the driver's seat. The control is in your hands.

C. *Combating depression with exercise.* I know it sounds absurd to ask yourself to exercise regularly when there are days you don't even have enough strength to get out of bed. But consider this: Exercise can build up our appetites and cause us to eat more food. Food is converted into energy so that we don't feel fatigued. When we decrease our fatigue factor, we also diminish the accompanying depression, irritability, confusion, and poor judgment.

D. *Birds of a Feather.* Join a support group composed of women who are undergoing your particular type of treatment or who have just finished. This is the time when swapping notes, jokes, stories, anecdotes, irritations, and outrages can be therapeutic, especially if the group is led by a licensed professional who is trained in breast cancer issues and will not allow negativity or gossip to get out of control or undermine your emotional well-being. If you aren't a "grouper," try some individual psychotherapy that will see you through until treatment is completed.

5. *I want a hundred percent guarantee against recurrence.* I don't blame you. So do I. Is there anyone who doesn't? We have bet our lives on the curative effects of chemotherapy and/or radiation. Wouldn't it be wonderful if our doctors could foresee the future?

Like most everything else in life, there are no guarantees. Each of us wonders, will the treatment "cure" me? If not, will it extend my life? Although the experts have good scientific evidence to support a *yes* answer in many cases, no one can ever guarantee it. That's why for our own emotional well being, it's so imperative that we understand the pros and cons of chemotherapy and radiation before we make our treatment decisions.

6. *Sad Sack Sex.* When we're in the midst of chemotherapy or radiation, sex isn't fun. It's a drag. In the first place, most of us are too tired to get in the mood. In the second place, many of us are not yet used to the change in our body appearance and this naturally affects our self-image and sexuality.

My best advice is: Tell it like it is. Be candid with your partner and say how you feel. There is no point in forcing yourself to have sex when all you really want to do is go to sleep, be left alone, or simply be held in your partner's arms. As the treatment draws to a close, you will find a reawakening of sexual interest and activity. If this doesn't happen, you will need to investigate whether other problems in the relationship are preventing sexual intimacy. That's when marriage or couples therapy is indicated. The important point to keep in mind is *there is no need to rush back into sex.* Most of us find that sexual desire returns when chemotherapy/radiation treatment ends. (Love, sex, and dating are discussed more thoroughly in Chapter Nine.)

Unnecessary/avoidable issues

1. *Scheduling appointments vs. disappointments.* Because the treatment can be lengthy and somewhat unpleasant, we owe it to ourselves to set up a schedule that is conve-

nient and will not cause disruptions elsewhere in our lives. For example, if we work at a traditional nine-to-five job, the best chemotherapy schedule is likely to be Friday afternoon, so that we have the weekend to recuperate, should we need it. Similarly, the best radiation schedule is prior to or immediately following work each day. I'm sure this is as obvious to you as it was to me. But our doctors and their office staffs don't always see it that way. They have a penchant for scheduling us in the middle of the week and/or the middle of the day. I have a theory as to why this is so. I call it "The Diner's Dilemma."

The Diner's Dilemma. Have you ever noticed when you go into an unfamiliar restaurant that unless you request a specific section or table you are likely to be seated facing the bathrooms? That's because the better tables are held for the regular customers. And reservations? Unless they know you, forget about being seated at the time you request. You get the leftover time slots.

Hypothetically, let's say you agree to dine in that restaurant five days a week for the next month or perhaps once every three weeks for the next six months. That would certainly make you a regular customer, right? Under those conditions, I bet you would get the table and reservation time you wish.

Why not apply this to our chemotherapy/radiation treatment? We are the regular customers. If we want a specific day and appointment time, we will be accommodated. If we can't get to first base with the front desk, all we have to do is talk to the management (our doctor).

HANNAH was a high school teacher who kept to herself. She didn't want to call attention to her chemotherapy by missing two days of school every few weeks in order to go for treatment.

The doctor's staff understood her need but couldn't switch treatment days from Wednesday to Friday because the doctor wasn't in the office on that day. They suggested she discuss the situation with him.

At first Hannah felt she had no right to ask the doctor to come in on his day off. But after mulling it over, she decided to let him know how she felt, even if nothing could be changed.

Good thing she did. It turned out that on Friday the doctor was in another office elsewhere in the city, and if she was willing to travel the distance (she was), he was perfectly willing to treat her there. She didn't have to miss a day or an hour of school and a problem was avoided.

Here's another example of scheduling that threatened to turn into disaster but was nipped in the bud. This one involved daily radiation treatments:

Ivy was an actress who never knew from one day to the next whether she would be going for an audition or working on a TV show. She required a flexible treatment schedule that allowed for last-minute changes.

The person in charge of setting up the schedule didn't like this arrangement at all. It was too much time and trouble to cater to Ivy's needs. So she told her that it couldn't be done. Ivy decided not to plead and argue. Instead, she saved her energy for a discussion with the doctor.

He agreed to her request, provided Ivy understood she would have to wait a little longer on the days when her appointment was "squeezed" into the schedule. She didn't mind waiting and was more than willing to make the tradeoff in order to have the freedom to pursue her career while she was undergoing treatment.

Both situations illustrate the fact that inconvenience and disappointment are not inevitable when scheduling our treatment. If our requests are not outrageous or impossible to satisfy, our doctors will make every effort to accommodate us.

One more thought before we leave this topic. All caring

doctors encourage their patients to engage in meaningful, constructive activities that will help take their minds off treatment. Therefore, if we require a schedule change in order to pursue a job or interest that gives our life a sense of control, purpose, pleasure, accomplishment, or well-being, we can be certain that our doctors will not want to throw a brick in our paths. When we let them know what makes us feel good about ourselves, most physicians will help us achieve it to the best of their ability.

   2. I never get to talk to the doctor for more than a few minutes. It is customary to have a consultation with the doctor each time we go for chemotherapy, or once a week if we are in radiation treatment. It would be nifty if they would set aside a good half-hour to *really* find out how we're doing and what we're worried about, instead of asking the cursory question, "Any problems?" while staring down at our chart instead of looking us straight in the eye. JASMIN, a chemotherapy patient, recalls:

> "I always got the impression that he was afraid I might actually say 'yes.' I never did say what was on my mind. I had plenty of questions all right, but I didn't feel he wanted to hear them. So each time I mumbled something to the effect that I was doing 'okay,' which wasn't exactly a lie but wasn't really the truth either, and shuffled out the door. He never pushed for more information, and I never offered it."

And that's how, with a little help from her doctor, Jasmin created an avoidable problem for herself. Believe me, we all do it in one way or another. I made the very same mistake. Years after my treatment ended, I acquired the courage to ask my radiation oncologist the questions I dared not ask during treatment. For some inexplicable reason, this time around he seemed friendlier and more open to my questions. This was very different from my original experience with him. So I began to wonder, did he really discourage my questions and hurry me out the door when I was in treatment? Or was I too afraid to hear answers that I might not like, so I didn't ask the questions, and then turned around and blamed him for the lack of communication? I'm not sure, but I think it's some of each.

Each of us can avoid this problem by letting our doctor know at the beginning of chemotherapy/radiation that we want extended consultations in order to clear up any concerns that may have aimlessly wandered into our thoughts.

3. The fragile doll syndrome. Don't be surprised when well-meaning family members, friends, employers, or co-workers find out you're in chemotherapy/radiation and react as if you're made of glass and about to shatter into a million pieces. Five minutes ago they were treating you like a good ole girl, and now suddenly you have been transformed into a fragile china doll or, worse, an invalid who is to be pitied.

They expect you to keel over and expire before their very eyes. It's enough to make you wonder if you shouldn't be more worried about your condition than you already are. You ask yourself, "Do they know something I don't know?" They would be shocked to find out that their "kindness" is emotionally crippling and not at all helpful.

The biggest danger, of course, is that some of us actually do buy into the fragile doll syndrome and become hopelessly depressed or convinced that we can't do anything for ourselves and that death is just around the corner.

4. The "you should be grateful" syndrome. Art Linkletter was right. People are funny. Not funny ha-ha. Funny peculiar. Some of them think that surviving breast cancer is such a miracle that we have no right to complain about the side effects of the chemotherapy/radiation. If we mention that we are losing our hair or have sores in our mouths from the chemotherapy, they will tell us how lucky we are to be alive and that we shouldn't be so ungrateful. The best solution is: Get rid of the bozos. But if the bozo in question happens to be our boss or a close family member, we may need to preserve the relationship. In that case, there are ways to do this without sacrificing our right to self-expression.

The most obvious is to refrain from telling him our feelings and, instead, share our concerns with those who are more cordial and receptive. Second, at the appropriate time, and in a polite way, give it back. When reason and dignity fail, benign retaliation gets positive results.

When LIZA told her sister-in-law, Nanette, that her radiation treatments made it difficult to swallow fibrous foods, Nanette's response was that she should be thrilled she didn't have to lose her breast or go through chemo, and this was a small price to pay. While this may have been true, it wasn't what Liza wanted (or needed) to hear.

The following week, Nanette told Liza how despondent she felt about approaching her fortieth birthday. Liza responded that she should be thrilled that she looked so good for her age and relieved that she could afford a face lift if necessary. Nanette felt hurt and said that Liza missed the point. Liza agreed and reminded her of their previous conversation about radiation treatment. Suddenly Nanette saw the light.

5. *Everyone has control of my life except me.* It ain't necessarily so . . . unless *you* make it so. When we are feeling miserable from the side effects of chemotherapy/radiation, we're certain we have no control over our lives. But if we use our initiative, we can control the quality and quantity of communication with our doctors, the choice of treatment, as well as our treatment times. We can also control the amount and type of interaction we have with any family member or friend. In fact, we have more

control over our lives than anyone else does. It's time we stop fighting this concept and start accepting it.

Are there psychological issues that are specific to chemotherapy and not radiation?

Yes. (For those wanting a more comprehensive discussion of chemotherapy than that offered in this chapter, please see Appendix A: Suggested Reading List.)

1. Chemotherapy tends to produce a greater number of short-term physical side effects that interfere with daily living and in turn cause a wide range of emotional reactions. For example, chemotherapy, unlike radiation, can make us physically ill for a couple of days or more following each treatment. This frequently disrupts our family life and work.

The chemotherapy process is often long and drawn out, lasting six months or a year. The temptation to quit is greater because the process is longer. (Radiation treatment lasts five to six weeks.) This temptation is compounded further by chronic fatigue, possible hair loss, weight fluctuation, infections, sores in the mouth, and peculiar tastes of foods. Last but not least, due to hormonal suppression of estrogen, we may experience menopausal symptoms such as hot flashes, cessation of menses, and loss of vaginal lubrication which makes sexual intercourse painful. All of these physical symptoms can cause psychological symptoms including: depression, low self-esteem, sexual inhibition, loss of sex drive, and fear of losing our partner.

2. The long-term side effects create other anxieties. For example, those of us who want to become pregnant are advised to wait several years after chemotherapy is com-

pleted before we conceive. This precaution is taken for two reasons. First, pregnancy causes hormonal fluctuations that can stimulate a recurrence of the cancer. Second, in order to reduce the risk of birth defects, it is imperative that no traces of toxic chemicals are left in the body. This "holding pattern" can be especially stressful if we are in our mid-to-late thirties, when we are more aware of our biological time clocks' ticking.

Even more anxiety-provoking is the possibility that we will become permanently sterile from the drugs, although irreversible infertility is rare in low-dose, short-term chemotherapy. In her book, *Coping with Chemotherapy,* author Nancy Bruning wrestles with this uncertainty:

> "The possibility of being sterile is not a major problem for me, since I have no overwhelming desire to have children. But it does seem odd—extending your own life in exchange for a potential child. At the moment it doesn't bother me—except that I do like to have options, whether I intend to exercise them or not, and this may have removed one of them. Now that having my own child may be out of the question, I sometimes feel a pang of regret. But who knows? I may be as fertile as I ever was, and it may never even be an issue."

3. Adjuvant chemotherapy/hormonal therapy has caused controversy. There are two issues in question. First, is the treatment really needed? Second, does it do more harm than good? Let's look at the pros and cons of each.

Is it really needed?
Pro: It acts as an insurance policy against possible recurrence by mopping up any stray cancer cells in the body, even though at present there is no measurable cancer to be found. If you believe in health, home, and car insurance, why not cancer insurance?

Con: Because there is nothing to measure, you have no way of knowing whether it's working. And if you don't know for sure that it *is,* why put yourself through the discomfort of the side effects? Plenty of women who don't get adjuvant chemo/hormonal therapy do fine and never have a recurrence.

Does it do more harm than good?

Pro: The short-term discomfort is worth the long-term survival, even though you will never know if it was the adjuvant chemo/hormonal therapy or your own body immune system that kept the cancer away.

Con: It's like killing a flea with a cannon! The potential long range side effects can include changes in the reproductive, digestive, and nervous system. And in extreme cases, chemotherapy drugs can cause cancer.

Conclusion: Yes, it does seem masochistic to volunteer for adjuvant chemo/hormonal therapy even though there is no concrete evidence that any cancer is still present. Yes, it is hard to justify putting ourselves through a myriad of miserable side effects when no one can tell for sure if it was needed or if it is working. Despite all of this, if your oncologist recommends it, I urge you to take it on faith that his educated guess is the right one.

And for those of us who need facts, not faith, here is the latest news: There is good evidence that adjuvant chemotherapy is beneficial to women who are less than 50 years old and who have positive lymph nodes. There is similar evidence that adjuvant hormonal therapy (tamoxifen) is beneficial to women who are over 50 years old and who have positive lymph nodes. Adjuvant chemotherapy and hormonal therapy *may possibly* benefit women with negative lymph nodes, regardless of age. The value of adjuvant chemotherapy in women who are over 50 years old and who have positive lymph nodes is questionable.

Are there psychological issues that are specific to radiation and not chemotherapy?

No doubt about it.

1. A lot of people think we are radioactive during and after our treatment. This is a myth. But if we believe it, or our friends and family do, our relationships are bound to come to a screeching halt. One patient got so tired of explaining to her co-workers that she wasn't radioactive that she assembled all of them in the conference room, turned off the lights, and announced, "You'll notice that I don't glow in the dark." They laughed nervously. She then flipped on the light switch and everyone began to discuss their fears of radiation and breast cancer. What a creative solution to an uncomfortable situation.

2. Radiation exposure. How much is too much? How come if it's not too much for me, it's too much for the technicians/nurses who are forever running out of the room before the radiation machine is turned on? I have to admit, their darting in and out of the treatment room didn't inspire my confidence or trust. But let's look at the other side of the coin. If the technicians didn't leave the room, they would be exposed to hours of radiation every day. Let's face it, that's a lot of radiation, and it's hard to blame them for being careful. But why must they run? It makes it seem so dangerous. Can't they calmly walk away?

I have it on good authority that the only reason they run is because we are uncomfortable in the pretzel-like positions they put us in, and they want to save us additional seconds of discomfort. They think they're doing us a favor! Conclusion? Once we discover the rationale for what appears to be strange or scary behavior, it becomes less worrisome and easier to tolerate. So talk to your tech when you don't understand a particular behavior or interaction between the two of you.

3. Have you noticed that the Magic Marker map on your chest resembles a wild rash or a frenzied follow-the-dot drawing? Mine was purple, like the kind you find on slabs of raw beef at the supermarket. In fact, my markings reminded me of the diagram charts of cows that you see

hanging on your butcher's wall. The technicians told me not to wash it off. I had heard of artistic temperament, but this was ridiculous. Did they mean no showers for the next month? No, I was told. Just wash carefully. (As opposed to what? Tossing the soap on the ceiling?)

Actually, none of it mattered in the long run because the very next night while I was asleep, I sweated the entire map of my chest onto my nightgown, sheets, and pillowcase, ruining them all. But worse than that was my fear that I had jeopardized my treatment by losing the magic markings. What if they couldn't find or follow the original dots?

Not to worry. The techs remarked the areas (called "ports"), this time in blue, my favorite color, and taped gauze over each dot so that the dye wouldn't run onto my clothes or bed linen. I also wore turtleneck sweaters (lucky for me it wasn't the summer months) to conceal the markings and gauze, especially near my collarbone and throat. It was a constant reminder of radiation treatment, but knowing it would end in a month made it bearable.

The way the people around us respond to "The Magic Marker Map" can be upsetting. MOLLIE unintentionally cleared out a public dressing room when she disrobed.

"I was near the end of the treatment and forgot about the red marking all over my chest. Suddenly I realized the women in the dressing room were staring at me. They were horrified by my appearance. First they moved across the room and then they quickly dressed and ran out. I felt like a leper. I wanted to call after them and say 'Come back, it's not contagious.' But I didn't. I put my clothes back on and cried all the way home. I knew what 'The Elephant Man' must have felt like."

Lesson to be learned? People get spooked very easily, especially strangers who don't know what's wrong with us and don't feel it's their place to ask. Reactions can be cruel and cause us unnecessary pain and suffering. Why go out and look for it? If you can't stand the heat, stay out of the kitchen. Or in this case, public dressing rooms.

Instead of "The Magic Marker Map," some doctors use the tattoo method in which a few tiny ink dots are strategically placed in the treatment area. The good news is the dots are barely noticeable. The bad news is they are yours forevermore because tattoos are permanent. Which one is preferable, a permanent souvenir of the occasion or a temporary graffiti exhibit on your chest? Most of us wind up feeling it's six of one and a half dozen of the other. However, if you have a decided preference, make it known to the radiation oncologist before you begin treatment.

4. The sci-fi look and sound of the equipment is frightening. (Are you sure this isn't Frankenstein's laboratory?) During the course of treatment, the machines will become more familiar and less threatening, but I don't expect you will ever grow to like them. Even now, years later, I find it hard to work up sincere enthusiasm when my radiation oncologist proudly shows me his new linear accelerator machine. I'm happy for him, but a little queasy in the stomach for me.

5. A frequent concern about the radiation technicians is: "How do I know if they're paying attention to what they're doing?" We feel at their mercy each day when they place us under the machine and administer the treatment. We may ask ourselves: "Did they get a good night's sleep, or are they so tired they accidentally pulled someone else's chart instead of mine? Are they concentrating on where to place my arm and head or are they thinking about their grocery lists? Do they realize how vulnerable I am to their words and actions?" To paraphrase the song, "They've Got My Whole World in Their Hands."

Our radiation technicians are acutely aware that we have these anxieties. If they don't broach the subject first, then they are waiting for us to mention it. And we would be foolish not to . . . if only to put our minds at ease. For example, one of the ways techs control for error is to cross-check each other. Frequently you have at least two people doing the setup and treatment. That way, if one tech makes a mistake, the other will see it and call it before any harm has occurred. Most of us find this comforting to know.

6. Our worst fears may be confirmed by iridium implants. At the end of treatment, some of us receive an external boost of radiation as out-patients and the rest of us receive iridium implants as in-patients. Who gets what is determined by the location of the excised cancerous tissue, but it is sometimes determined by whether our doctor has the newer external boost machine. Mine didn't. So off I went to the hospital for the implants, where the first thing that greeted me was a big sign posted on my door warning all passers-by (and those foolhardy enough to dare enter my room) that radioactivity lurked behind the door. Honestly, all that was missing was a skull and crossbones. Don't worry, I was told, it's just hospital policy.

Next, I was advised that it would be best if my visitors limited their time with me to no more than an hour a day in order to avoid radiation exposure. They had to sit at least ten feet away from my bed. And they shouldn't be pregnant or under eighteen. But don't worry, I was told, it's just hospital policy. I decided to tell my friends exactly what I had been told. And guess what? They decided to stay away. Who could blame them? Iridium implants give a whole new meaning to the song "You Light Up My Life."

Slowly the nurses began to appear (and mostly disappear). They wore strange little counting machines pinned to their uniforms. I was told they were radiation counters, but not to worry, it was just hospital policy. Be that as it may, they never stayed to chat or find out how I was feeling. They tossed the meal trays into the room as if I played catcher for the Dodgers. They avoided me as much as they could. I felt rejected and abandoned. Those were the loneliest forty-eight hours I have ever known.

If I had been given the choice, I would have preferred an external boost, even though it meant going for a longer time. It appears to me to be less psychologically stressful. And there are no pits or scars left from the implant rods. If your doctor gives you a choice between the two, you may want to weigh the time factor against the emotional factor before you make your final decision.

7. What about the end result? A side effect of the final product is that your untreated breast will age naturally and droop over time, while the treated breast, due to tissue change, will remain firmer and more erect. Some of us find this amusing while others find it annoying. Then there is a third group who are so pleased with their unexpected breast uplift that they want to have the other breast irradiated too! This whole business of one breast growing old while the other stays young reminds me of the Oscar Wilde novel, *The Picture of Dorian Gray,* in which only the painting grows old. If this "one hung low" phenomenon distresses you, a surgical breast uplift can be performed on the untreated breast.

One final thought on chemotherapy/radiation blues and how to chase them away. Learning how to do our own guided imagery and self-hypnosis can help us relax whenever the treatment or the side effects make us anxious, stressed, fatigued, or depressed. There are some excellent commercial tapes available or we may wish to have one made specifically for us by a licensed psychotherapist who is also a certified hypnotherapist. We need to make sure the person we choose has proper credentials and is known to our doctor.

Summary

Chemotherapy and radiation have vastly different physical side effects, but share many similar psychological side effects.

A. *Universal unavoidable issues include:*
- fear that the treatment will do more harm than good
- fear of the unknown
- feeling fatigued and depressed
- lack of interest in sex
- wanting a hundred percent guarantee against recurrence

B. *Unnecessary/avoidable issues include:*
- communication problems with medical staff (especially in scheduling treatment days and times)
- unavailability of the doctor to speak with us
- the fragile doll syndrome (when family, friends, coworkers treat us as if we're going to break into a million pieces at any moment)
- the you-should-be-grateful syndrome (the flip side of the fragile doll syndrome. This time the message is "you should be strong, stoic, and silent")
- everyone has control over my life except me

Specific radiation complaints that create emotional havoc include:
- the myth that we are radioactive
- fear of radiation exposure—ours
- fear of radiation exposure—theirs (family, friends, and medical staff)
- the indignity of the process (having our chest and back "mapped out" with brightly colored Magic Marker that can't be washed off for a month)
- trying to find clothing that conceals "the map"
- living with permanent dots tattooed to our chest
- the frightening sci-fi look and sound of the machines and equipment
- feeling at the mercy of the technicians who provide treatment
- fixed and rigid schedule of treatment

- feeling exhausted
- the impersonal once-a-week-once-over by the radiation oncologist
- feeling abandoned and rejected in the hospital when the iridium implants are in your breast
- cosmetic changes in breast appearance

Specific chemotherapy complaints that produce psychological turmoil include:
- feeling physically ill for several days or weeks following each treatment
- disruption of family life
- interruption in work schedule
- long drawn-out process lasting months, sometimes years
- temptation to quit
- hair loss
- weight fluctuations
- mouth sores
- peculiar taste of food
- menopausal symptoms
- sexual inhibitions
- loss of sex drive
- fear of losing our partner
- implications for future pregnancy
- the adjuvant chemotherapy controversy

Learning to do our own guided imagery and self-hypnosis can help relax us whenever chemotherapy/radiation side effects make us anxious, stressed, fatigued, or depressed.

Scheduling special treats at regular and frequent intervals can help make the chemotherapy/radiation routine more tolerable. We can actually condition a positive response to a negative experience by rewarding ourselves for having endured it.

CHAPTER EIGHT

Getting Back

to Business:

Career and

Job Issues

*I*t's your absolute right to keep your treatment for breast cancer a private matter, one that is not open for office discussion. Having said that, let me add that if you succeed, you deserve to be on the first page of "Ripley's Believe It Or Not."

It is the rare business or company that doesn't have a grapevine. So if you are planning to withhold this information, you may be in for a big surprise.

Let's take a look at why many of us feel the need to keep our treatment for breast cancer a secret from our employers, employees and/or co-workers:

"They will think I'm sickly, perhaps dying, and then use that as a reason to avoid me, or get me to quit my job."

"I will be treated like an invalid and made to feel that I'm different from the others."

"They will talk behind my back, maybe even make fun of me."

"They will speculate about my sex life."

"They will ask questions that I'm not ready to discuss or don't even have the answers to."

"They don't really give a damn about me or how all of this affects my life. They're curious in a ghoulish way . . . as if they're slowing down the car to get a good look at an accident."

Our need for privacy doesn't have to conflict with our co-workers' curiosity, concern, or even nosiness. In fact, sometimes by keeping our treatment a secret from the office staff, we wind up creating the very situation and emotional discomfort we were desperately trying to avoid.

BETSY was unusually attractive, with long, flaming red hair. She told no one at the office of her diagnosis and impending surgery, and used her summer vacation to recuperate from the mastectomy and begin chemo. When she returned to work, she wore a short red wig. Everyone was stunned. Naturally, they wanted to know what prompted her to cut off her beautiful red hair. Betsy was flustered and couldn't think of a credible answer. This piqued everyone's curiosity even further. Then, when she missed work every other Friday, the rumors began to fly. The consensus was it must be a terminal case of cancer. In reality, Betsy's breast cancer was not terminal, but her mysterious behavior led people to jump to the worst conclusion.

What happened to Betsy was an avoidable problem. It didn't have to happen to her and it certainly doesn't have to happen to you.

Disclosing the specifics of our treatment to the gang at work requires a combination of savvy and psychological awareness. Don't worry, you don't need the expertise of Dr. Joyce Brothers to successfully pull this off. There are seven basic factors to keep in mind: who, what, when, where, why, how, and how much.

1. *Who* do you tell and *why?*

A. *Your boss???* All things being equal, it's generally a wise idea to take your boss into your confidence since he is in the position to make your life easier during your course of treatment and recovery. Anything that you can do to facilitate having an easier time of it is definitely in your best interest. Because your boss is also responsible for your attendance, as well as the quantity and quality of your job performance, you have more to gain by disclosing this information than you do by withholding it. This is particularly significant if you need or want to take some sick time.

Even if your boss is a louse, you're still better off letting him know what's going on, if only to prevent him from feeling foolish should the higher-ups ask questions about you, your health, or your absences. Also, if other people at work know and your boss doesn't, it's bound to create a lot of ill will between the two of you when he finds out.

Although I advocate honesty as the best policy for coping effectively with breast cancer, I don't recommend that you volunteer your diagnosis or treatment to *prospective* employers. If they ask, I urge you to tell the truth. Incidentally, if they do ask and you don't tell the truth and then later they catch you (and there is a good chance they will), that may be grounds for immediate dismissal.

B. *Your employees???* Maybe. If your employees have the attitude "while the cat's away, the mice will play," you're probably better off not saying anything to them. On the other hand, if they are dedicated workers who won't take advantage of you or the situation, why not share this information? For one thing, it makes you more human and less "bossy." For another, your employees are going to notice your absences eventually and wonder what's going on. And as we have already seen, when we don't make any information available, there is a tendency for others to suspect the worst.

C. *Your co-workers???* Only tell the ones you genuinely like. The advantage of having this type of alliance with your favorite co-workers is they will protect you from the gossipmongers. When anyone else in the office raises a question or makes a comment, they will run interference. There is absolutely no good reason to take into your confidence any co-worker you dislike.

2. *What* do you say and *how much?*

Say as much as your business associates need to know in order to keep the office running smoothly. No more, no less. Keep it straightforward and honest. If they want more information, they will ask. Most people will not pry for details unless you volunteer them first. When questions come up that are related to your breast cancer treatment, it's your option to disclose the information or decline further details. But if the questions relate to your ability to perform your job during the treatment/recovery time, try to answer them to the best of your knowledge. Should you begin to feel pressured, politely stop the conversation. You can always continue it later when you feel less stressed.

If your business associates ask in what way they can be of help, for heaven's sake, tell them. This is no time to be bashful (or any other of the seven dwarfs). At the very least, you need their understanding and emotional support since it will take you some time to return to feeling like your old self. But more than that, there may be job duties that are too exhausting for you to perform right now that they are willing, if not happy, to cover. *It's okay to request a lighter workload during treatment and recovery. It doesn't mean that you are lazy or an invalid.*

Even if you aren't receiving chemotherapy or radiation, you will still need to be careful not to pull your arm, shoulder, and back muscles on the surgery side. So ask for assistance instead of straining and spraining.

3. *When* do you disclose the information?

Do you tell the folks at work what's going on before you go for treatment? Do you wait until they notice a change, begin asking questions, and/or are chatting among themselves? Or do you finish up and then tell them after the fact?

A. *Before???*

Here are the advantages:

1. It's one less ball that you need to juggle. If you disclose the information right away, you don't have to make up stories about where you're going and what you're doing. Besides, if you're not a good liar, you'll do a crummy job of it and someone is bound to get wise.

2. The sooner you tell, the sooner you can get emotional support and empathy. This prevents unnecessary misunderstandings that lead to avoidable problems.

3. If there is someone at work who was successfully treated for breast cancer and wants to be a support system or a role model, it gives both of you the opportunity to explore this possibility.

Here is the disadvantage:

1. You may have to fend off annoying questions for a longer period of time. But since this is a skill that you will also need to acquire in your nonbusi-

ness relationships, it will actually give you needed practice.

B. *During???*

The advantages are exactly the same as *Before*.

Here are the disadvantages:

1. If they figure it out for themselves prior to your decision to tell them, they may feel hurt that you didn't take them into your confidence sooner. They may also feel guilty because they would have been more understanding and cooperative had they known.

2. It will be harder to quell office gossip because any factual information you now give them will be mixed in with a lot of misinformation and rumor. Once the cat is out of the bag, it's hard to coax it back in again.

C. *After???*

Here is the advantage:

1. The "bite the bullet" crowd at the office will admire your courage and spirit for having braved such a trauma in secrecy.

Here are the disadvantages:

1. It's a long time to go without emotional support and empathy from your business associates. It's also self-punitive to deny yourself the care and concern from your colleagues.

2. Because you were so secretive, there may be a feeling in the office that this is just the tip of the iceberg. The staff may incorrectly assume that you know a lot more than you're telling.

4. *How* and *where* do you break the news?

Once again, there are no hard and fast rules. Do what is most comfortable. Some of us are more secure with a face-to-face discussion, while many prefer a telephone conversation, and still others want a third person (usually a spouse) to act as the intermediary. All are acceptable.

If you decide to have a third person act as your telephone intermediary when initially breaking the news to your employer, make sure you discuss beforehand exactly what you want him to say and not say. If you feel anxious about this, write out a brief script and rehearse it together.

Similarly, if your boss or someone else at the office is going to be your go-between for the rest of the employees, be specific as to what you do and don't want disclosed to the staff. Don't forget to include your wishes with regard to phone calls and visits.

If you choose an in-person meeting you will need to decide beforehand whether you want to do this in a group format or individually. Naturally, there are advantages and disadvantages to both.

Group meeting advantages: It saves time and energy because everyone hears the same information at the same time. If you believe in the old saying "There's safety in numbers," then you will find that a group meeting provides less chance for your information to be misinterpreted, distorted, or misunderstood.

Group meeting disadvantages: A group meeting doesn't allow for individual differences. It's very unlikely that you feel exactly the same way about each person in the office, and even more unlikely that you would talk to each person in precisely the same way. In other words, the group meeting is less personal and personalized.

Individual meeting advantages: You can tailor your discussion with each person allowing for the degree of intimacy and friendship you desire, how much he wants to know, and what, if any, assistance you will be needing from this person during your treatment and/or recuperation.

You allow for a stronger bond of friendship to develop between the two of you.

You can dispel any myths or fears the person may have.

Individual meeting disadvantages: Depending on the number of people in your office, it can get unwieldy and stressful. If it's a few people, fine. But a half dozen or more are unmanageable, tedious, and much too emotionally draining.

Individual meetings result in individual interpretations of your diagnosis and prognosis. Each person hears what is said in his own unique way . . . which may or may not be what you said.

Combining individual and group meetings: Rather than choosing one or the other (group vs. individual meetings), you may want to consider a combination of the two. For example, try individual meetings with one or two key members of the office and a group meeting with the rest of the staff.

Here's how three patients successfully avoided being the target of office gossip by disclosing just enough information to keep everyone informed, while simultaneously safeguarding their right to privacy.

ERIN: "On my first day back at work following the surgery, I asked my favorite co-workers to join me for a potluck lunch on Friday. They knew I had been on sick leave for several weeks but didn't know why. During the course of lunch, I told them about my mastectomy and immediate reconstruction. No further treatment was needed and, God willing, I had seen the last of my breast cancer. Before they could ask questions, I said that I really didn't want to talk about the details yet . . . if ever. They appreciated my honesty. A couple were flattered that I took them into my confidence.

I'm glad I waited until it was over to tell the people at work. They understood and never pried or gossiped. But I think if I had waited past that first week, there would have been some hot rumors flying around."

PATRICE: "I went into the hospital the day after I was diagnosed. Terrified, I telephoned my boss and told her what was going on and that I would be out from work for a few weeks. She was wonderful. She asked if I wanted anyone else to know. I said it was okay for her to tell the rest of the women in our department. She took care of the whole office thing for me. She broke the news to my co-workers while I was in the hospital. They sent flowers and, once a day, someone from the office called to check up on how I was doing. I preferred that to being bombarded with phone calls and visitors. But the best part of it was that the shock value was over by the time I returned to work.

I know for me it was a very good idea to have my boss act as my intermediary. It saved me from a lot of explanation and awkwardness on my first week back at the job."

RANDI: "I knew I was going to be fatigued from treatment and would be arriving an hour late to work each morning because that was the earliest radiation appointment I could get. I didn't particularly want to tell my twelve employees that I had breast cancer, but I also realized that if I didn't say something, they would be wondering about my peculiar coming and goings.

So I organized a brief coffee break in which we put all the phones on hold and I told them what happened and what I was anticipating in the way of treatment. I also told them there would be times when I would be open to questions and conversations on the subject and there would be other times when I would be closed . . . so they shouldn't take it personally if I wasn't in the mood to talk. We discussed what I wanted and needed from each of them, including what felt supportive and what didn't, so that they could assist me in making my treatment and recovery time more relaxing and less stressful.

It worked beautifully. I really believe that because I was

open and honest with my employees, they were more
cooperative and supportive of their boss."

As you can see, there is no one right way to disclose
your diagnosis/treatment. Nor is it mandatory that you
disclose any information at all. If you work in a setting
where you rarely see the same people more than once or
twice a month, you may have no reason or need to tell
them anything. The point is this: The best way to fuel the
fire of office gossip is to tell a lie or withhold the truth
about your treatment. Conversely, the best way to quench
the thirst for office gossip is to voluntarily share a small
amount of honest and factual information about your
situation. It makes the people in your office feel that you
trust them and, as a result, they will invariably prove
themselves worthy of this belief.

How do you handle office prejudice and fear?

Prejudice and fear grow out of ignorance. Education
and information are our best weapons. If and when you
decide to disclose your treatment to the various people in
your office, you may also want to have some basic pamphlets handy and available for those who express an interest in knowing more about breast cancer. The National
Cancer Institute publishes easy-to-read material that specifically addresses breast cancer myths and fears. (See
Appendix A: Suggested Reading.)

If you work for a large organization, you may want to
arrange with the personnel department to invite a breast
cancer specialist from the community to come in on an
employee lunch hour to discuss how early detection of
breast cancer can save your life. It would be advantageous
to encourage male employees to attend. After all, many

men are married to women who, unfortunately, may one day be diagnosed with this disease.

Some folks are so stubborn that no amount of education and personal interaction seems to make a dent in their skulls. Their attitude is "Don't confuse me with facts." If you find yourself up against this type of character or situation, just walk away. If education doesn't work, ignore the ignorant.

Occasionally office prejudice and fear turn into job discrimination, within your own company or when looking for a new position.

For example, I counseled a distressed woman who was teaching at a vocational school at the time she was diagnosed. The day after she told the owner, he fired her, explaining: "Cancer comes from putting out bad vibes and you might contaminate me." (Ironically, it was the lawsuit for wrongful dismissal and the adverse publicity that followed that contaminated him.)

In another situation, one of my patients was diagnosed with breast cancer during the probationary period of her new job. She was immediately discharged without health insurance coverage. Unemployed and uninsured, she ferreted out low-fee medical treatment. Perhaps the company that fired her was within their legal rights, but you have to wonder about their sense of decency.

Another woman, at age sixty-two, was asked by her employer to put in for an early retirement after she was treated for breast cancer. She wasn't ready to retire and resented being pushed out of her job. The company was within their legal rights and didn't much care that the patient's self-worth and self-esteem had suffered a second cruel blow in less than a year.

Anyone who tells you job discrimination doesn't exist for breast cancer patients must be living on Mars.

So what's a girl to do? You have three options:

• Accept the role of victim. Keep your feelings locked up and convince yourself that they were right to fire you. Tell yourself you deserved what you got (in which case you won't be needing this book or wanting to read it).

• Pick yourself up, dust yourself off, and make a fresh start. Vent the hurt and anger with family, friends, support groups, and/or in individual psychotherapy. And then get back out there and find yourself a job that is more gratifying and fulfilling than the one you left or didn't get. Please keep in mind that most employers are not cancerphobic or prejudiced. You will find the right match if you give yourself a fair chance.

But what if you really love your job and are certain that you can't find a similar one, or if you do, you will have to take a substantial salary cut? What can you do then?

• Fight back! If you have the energy to stick with it, you stand a good chance of winning. Fighting back is serious business and a healthy outlet for frustration and anger— provided it is channeled effectively. Here is a list of *Dos* and *Don'ts* to help you fight effectively:

1. *Do* contact the company president and politely but firmly tell him what has occurred and that you intend to pursue the matter further. Leave it ambiguous as to what "further" actually means. This gives him a chance to make good and straighten out the situation. Be pleasant. I'm a firm believer in the adage: "You can catch more flies with honey than with vinegar." If that fails:

2. *Do* contact your local media (television, radio, and newspaper). A particularly good contact is the consumer advocate reporter. If you can whet the reporter's appetite to investigate your story, you're practically home free. Frequently when companies are subjected to the questions of an investigative reporter, they back down fast and settle the matter privately, before they receive undesirable pub-

licity and public condemnation. If that doesn't bring satisfaction:

3. *Do* contact an attorney, preferably one who has earned a reputation for handling civil rights cases and/or women's rights. You will be told whether you have a winable case. If you do, the attorney's fee will be a percentage of whatever settlement you receive.

The *Don't* list includes:

1. *Don't* threaten, harass, and/or harangue your former employer. (I don't care if they're cretins and deserve every word of your wrath. This is a good way to make yourself appear in the wrong, even though you are in the right.)

2. *Don't* bad-mouth your former employer to prospective employers. (I'm sure you know a grapevine exists in every profession, field, and business. And even though the prospective employer may love to hear dirt about the competitor, you can be certain that he is also wondering how much of it is true, and whether you are a troublemaker who will wind up turning against his firm as well.)

3. *Don't* try to involve other employees in your battle. You will be putting your friends in an uncomfortable situation where they are forced to choose sides. Since they need their jobs to pay their bills, you will find yourself in a no-win position. (This issue has enough merit to stand on its own; you don't need a lynch mob to prove your point.)

Because job discrimination feels so humiliating and embarrassing, it becomes all too easy to fall into the "victim" trap. If you opt for this choice, you will carry around feelings of depression, anger, and shame. The only truly effective coping strategies in this situation are to constructively fight back or "pick yourself up, dust yourself off, and make a fresh start."

Sometimes the difficulty isn't with our employer, but with our employee health insurance coverage:

What health insurance problems should we be prepared for?

It's a shame that such a question still needs to be asked. But it does. And since your health insurance company calls the tune, it's important that you know all the lyrics. The typical types of health insurance problems are knowable, solvable, and sometimes even avoidable. So here we go:

If your coverage is relatively new, there will be an investigation to determine whether you were previously diagnosed, and are now trying to pull a fast one by getting your new health insurance company to foot the bill for treatment. Don't tear your hair out trying to argue logic with your insurance company. It just won't work. The only language they understand is 'computerspeak.' The problem will get resolved, but very, very slowly. It may take many months before you or any of your doctors receive payment. The best way to expedite the matter is to get the name of the supervisor handling your claim and initiate weekly, leading up to daily, conversations with him until all the bills are paid.

Also, it's a good idea for you and your doctor's billing service to keep each other informed of your progress so that each doesn't think the other one is taking care of it, only to discover no one is.

If you change jobs, you may not be able to find another private health insurance carrier willing to cover you. Or if they do, you may have a long waiting period in which you must be symptom- and treatment-free before your new health insurance company will cover you for cancer. Health Maintenance Organizations (frequently referred to as H.M.O.s) such as Kaiser-Permanente currently do not have such exclusions under their group plans. Consequently, many patients decide to join H.M.O.s for that reason and especially if they have no secondary health insurance coverage through a spouse.

If you are considering leaving your job, make sure your prospective employer will give you full medical coverage. You absolutely cannot afford to be without adequate health insurance, which means your policy needs to include cancer coverage. Needless to say, you would be foolish to go without any health insurance at all.

Some women opt to convert their group coverage to an individual plan when they leave their jobs. This usually turns out to be a very expensive proposition and the coverage is skimpier than the group policy. But when you have no choice, it's better than nothing.

There are a number of organizations working on health insurance reform for cancer patients. The one that is most appropriate for our needs is the National Alliance of Breast Cancer Organizations, headquartered in New York City. (Individual memberships are welcomed.) It may not be a club that any of us *aspire* to join. But it sure is one that we all *need* to join. (See Appendix C: Organizations of Interest).

Summary

When it comes to the office, to tell or not to tell, that is the question. There are pros and cons to consider before reaching final decisions.

No one wants to be the target of office gossip. Our need for privacy doesn't have to conflict with our co-workers' curiosity, concern, or even nosiness.

Disclosing the specifics of our treatment to the office staff requires a combination of savvy and psychological awareness. It also includes knowing:

- *Who* to tell and *why*.
- *What* to say and *how much*.
- *When* to disclose this information.
- *How* and *where* to break the news.

The best way to handle fellow employees' prejudice and fear is through education, information, and discussion.

When job discrimination does occur, we have three choices:

- Accept the role of victim.
- Pick ourselves up, dust ourselves off, and make a fresh start.
- Fight back in a constructive and effective way.

Should we need to fight back, there are strategic *Dos* and *Don'ts* that can psychologically strengthen or weaken our position.

The typical types of health insurance problems we may encounter are knowable, solvable, and, sometimes, even avoidable.

- If our coverage is new, there will be an investigation to determine a preexisting condition or diagnosis.
- If the insurance reimbursements are not paid in a timely manner, get the name of the supervisor handling the claim, and initiate weekly contact until the bill is paid.
- Keep the doctor's billing service informed of any and all contact you have with the insurance com-

pany, so that both of you are in sync and not duplicating efforts.

- If we change jobs we may find ourselves uninsurable or have a long waiting period before we are eligible for breast cancer coverage. Our options include converting our group policy into individual coverage or joining an H.M.O. group plan.

Love, Sex,

Dating, and

Marriage

*W*hen I do interviews, the most popular question asked is: "After breast cancer surgery, who has an easier sexual adjustment—the married woman or the single/divorced woman?" If you guessed married women, guess again.

The quality of the relationship between you and your partner is the key to sexual adjustment, not whether you are married, single, divorced, or widowed. When the quality of the relationship is good or excellent, married women usually have an easier sexual adjustment than single women. However, when the quality of the relationship is mediocre or poor, married women usually have a much more difficult time of it than single women.

Having to cope with your husband's problems as well as your own can be overwhelming at a time like this. In other words, *a lousy relationship is worse than no relationship at all.* I'm convinced this is true for all women, with or without breast cancer. I suspect we all know this in our heart of hearts, although many fight hard not to admit it. What breast cancer does is give us the opportunity to find out whether we picked a peach or a lemon.

Do most women find sex intimidating after breast cancer?

Yes. But there are ways to reduce the embarrassment and make it less emotionally difficult. And that's what this chapter is about. Sexual adjustment following breast cancer treatment is delicate, regardless of your marital status. There are the avoidable problems such as waiting to see if he'll make the first move and trying to figure out what it means if he does or doesn't (and what we can do to avoid falling into this trap). And there are the universal/unavoidable issues such as the awkwardness of undressing in front of your partner for the first time. (It's like being a teenager all over again.)

Whatever your issues may be, please know they are solvable. Love and sex after breast cancer don't have to be traumatic or create emotional upheaval unless you ignore your feelings until they run out of control.

If the relationship was good B.C. (Before Cancer), it will be good A.D. (After Diagnosis). In fact, some couples insist that breast cancer treatment made them closer and more intimate because it forced them to talk more openly about sex, what feels good, and what hurts.

CANDY: "After my mastectomy, the right side of my chest was sore. We had two choices available to us. One was to give up sex until the incision healed, which didn't appeal to either one of us. The other was to invent new ways to make love without putting weight on that part of my chest. They say that necessity is the mother of invention. It certainly was for us."

On the other hand, if the relationship wasn't so terrific B.C., then it is likely that the feelings about your breast and the cancer will become yet another one of the unresolved issues between you A.D.

RITA: "I never enjoyed sex with Carl. I would do it more or less to make him happy. So you would think I'd be pleased that since the surgery, he doesn't bother me for sex any more. But it upsets me that he's lost interest. I feel like I'm not feminine enough for him now."

The quality of Rita's relationship with Carl was poor before her surgery. Sex wasn't pleasurable. It was an obligation and a charade. This couple first needs to develop an honest relationship with each other before they contemplate sexual activity.

The bottom line is this: Whatever existed between the two of you B.C. is what's going to exist between the two of you A.D.—only more so. If it was good, it will get better. If it was bad, it will get worse . . . unless you do something about it.

What can you do to improve on the existing relationship or prevent it from deteriorating any further?

Learn how to communicate more effectively. In order to have a quality relationship, you need good communication. Both of you must care about what the other person says and feels. If you talk with each other on a daily basis, romance and sex will follow.

RUTH was certain that her mastectomy would lead to divorce since she and her husband, Ben, rarely talked or expressed feelings to one another. Although they loved each other, Ben's affairs with other women had nearly wrecked their marriage in years past and Ruth suspected he would soon begin to repeat this behavior. Rather than waiting to see if her instincts were right, she and Ben came for help.

I recommended they begin a daily exercise consisting of a half-hour of conversation with each other. They were free to talk about whatever each was feeling or thinking. Although they had some initial resistance to this assignment, calling it foolish and not being able to find a time that they could stick to, they finally settled into the groove and discovered that they enjoyed each other's conversation. The talking created intimacy; the intimacy created romance and sex. Conversely, they found that when they sloughed off "talking" for a few nights, the relationship began to drift apart.

If you or your partner has lost interest in sex, you need to talk about why, and find out what the two of you can do to improve the situation.

You may think his/your lack of sexual desire has to do with your physical appearance. I'm not saying this doesn't ever happen, but frankly it's the exception and not the rule. More frequently the reasons for losing sexual interest are: *depression* because one or both of you feels powerless to help you, or to change the situation; *anger* that the disease has interrupted your lives and current plans; *fear* of death, dying, and coming to grips with mortality, yours and his. It's difficult to feel amorous when there are so many negative emotions competing for his/your energy.

Do something romantic together like going for a walk in the woods, a picnic, or a sailboat ride. Find time to be with each other and plan it so that you have no intrusions. A weekend for two without kids and phones is perfect.

Who should initiate sex for the first time following surgery?

This is a toughie. For romantic reasons—him. For medical reasons—you. For traditional relationships—him. For liberated relationships—you. In other words, the needs of the relationship dictate the answer. If you have a nontraditional relationship in which you are assertive and independent, it makes sense that you will initiate sex when you feel ready. On the other hand, if you are a traditionalist, you will probably feel more comfortable if your partner makes the initial overture. My philosophy is: It's an avoidable problem. Don't turn it into a test of love or you will have a major avoidable problem on your hands. It doesn't matter who makes the first move, just so long as one of you does . . . and while you're still young enough to remember what to do, and how to do it!

Jokes aside, a more important question than who initiates sex is *why now?* Is it because both of you really want to make love? Or are you doing it out of obligation because you think your partner expects it? If the answer is the latter, you need to be talking to each other more, and worrying about sex less.

If you're curious as to whether the quality of your relationship with your partner is helping or hindering your emotional and psychological recovery from breast cancer, take this quiz and find out.

Relationship Quiz

Please check the column that best describes how you feel.

	ALWAYS	USUALLY	SOMETIMES	RARELY	NEVER
1. I am interesting.	☐	☐	☐	☐	☐
2. My partner is interesting.	☐	☐	☐	☐	☐
3. I am attractive.	☐	☐	☐	☐	☐
4. My partner is attractive.	☐	☐	☐	☐	☐
5. I am likable.	☐	☐	☐	☐	☐
6. My partner is likable.	☐	☐	☐	☐	☐
7. I am considerate.	☐	☐	☐	☐	☐
8. My partner is considerate.	☐	☐	☐	☐	☐
9. I can be trusted.	☐	☐	☐	☐	☐

10. My partner can be trusted. ☐ ☐ ☐ ☐ ☐

11. I am *willing* to express my feelings. ☐ ☐ ☐ ☐ ☐

12. My partner is *willing* to express his feelings. ☐ ☐ ☐ ☐ ☐

13. I am *able* to express my feelings. ☐ ☐ ☐ ☐ ☐

14. My partner is *able* to express his feelings. ☐ ☐ ☐ ☐ ☐

15. I am a good listener. ☐ ☐ ☐ ☐ ☐

16. My partner is a good listener. ☐ ☐ ☐ ☐ ☐

17. I can compromise without holding a grudge. ☐ ☐ ☐ ☐ ☐

18. My partner can compromise without holding a grudge. ☐ ☐ ☐ ☐ ☐

19. Before breast cancer, I enjoyed sex with my partner. ☐ ☐ ☐ ☐ ☐

20. Since my breast cancer, I enjoy sex with my partner. ☐ ☐ ☐ ☐ ☐

Scoring

Please score 5 points for each answer you marked AL-WAYS, 4 points for USUALLY, 3 points for SOMETIMES, 2 points for RARELY, 1 point for NEVER.

80–100: The quality of your relationship is excellent, and you are very unlikely to experience serious relationship problems as a result of your breast cancer treatment. Whatever you're doing is working, so keep on doing it!

60–79: The quality of your relationship is good, but could stand some polishing. Any serious problems you experience in the relationship as a result of your breast cancer treatment are easily solved through discussion. If you and your partner are willing to go for some brief psychotherapy, that would be helpful.

40–59: The quality of your relationship isn't so hot, and you probably didn't need this quiz to figure it out. The breast cancer problems are the tip of the iceberg. Get some professional help now, with or without your partner, before things get worse.

20–39: You are in a toxic relationship. Get out now, while you still have the emotional strength to pack your suitcase. I'm serious about this. Stay with a friend or relative. There are deep problems between the two of you that are already making your breast cancer treatment/recovery very difficult, if not close to impossible. (I realize this is easier said than done for a woman with two or three children and limited means.)

A few words about your score: If your overall score was high, but you answered NEVER or RARELY to *any* of the questions, it is an indicator of trouble down the road. For now, it's not important whether the cause of the trouble is you, your partner, or both of you. What is important is that you have identified a problem area that needs to be solved before it begins to affect other aspects of the relationship. If you can't, or don't know how to resolve the problem on your own, get some professional help. If you were a car, you would take yourself to a mechanic and have the squeak or rattle checked out. Why not do the same for your relationship? Check it out with a psychotherapist.

If your partner wants out, when is he likely to exit?

If your husband/lover wants to end the relationship, he will do it either at the time of diagnosis (which means he was getting ready to split anyway and had one foot out the door), or he will wait until after you complete your treatment (which means he thinks you're healthy and it's safe to move on without guilt). Rarely will a partner end the relationship while his wife/girlfriend is in chemotherapy or radiation treatment. Why? It's too guilt-provoking to leave your mate when she's down and out. The oddballs who do split in the middle of treatment are the ones who have no pangs of guilt or conscience. They would have left anyhow, at the first sign of discomfort or inconvenience. Your illness simply speeded up the process.

So what does all of this mean? It means that many of us won't have the benefit of a monogamous relationship during our treatment and recovery from breast cancer. We will have to go through the process without a spouse/lover in our lives. This is not necessarily tragic. In fact, in certain instances, it is actually a blessing.

What are the potential problems for the woman who is dating?

1. *To tell or not to tell on the first date, that is the question.* Some say it's the only way to go, while others guarantee it will scare the guy off. Weigh both sides of the issue and decide for yourself.

The advantages are:

A. You find out right away if he's a cancerphobe and save yourself a lot of heartache. (If he gasps, faints, or brings the date to a swift close, you know you've got a cancerphobe on your hands.)

B. It makes it real easy for him to tell you about his traumatic/life-threatening illness. (It seems as if every man has an important illness that he wants to discuss with a woman who won't be scared away.)

CAMILLE had been through a number of relationships that hadn't worked out. She had no more patience left for another relationship that was doomed from the start. So she decided to tell Mark, on their first date, of her mastectomy and breast reconstruction. His reaction was refreshing and unexpected. He immediately confided in her that he was diabetic and that it complicated his life to the point that he often wondered if any woman would be seriously interested in him as a mate. Camille was and still is.

C. It immediately sets the stage for an open, honest relationship.

The disadvantages are:

A. It's too much, too soon. It's a heavy trip to lay on a guy who isn't even sure that he wants to see you for a second date. And before the evening is over, you may have similar reservations about him for an entirely different set of reasons.

B. He may think you're apologizing for yourself or offering him a disclaimer because you see yourself as "defective merchandise" or "damaged goods."

C. You may get rejection instead of a round of applause. Do you have the ego strength and self-esteem to handle it without becoming depressed? When you play with matches, you can get burned.

BOBBIE: "I expected a pat on the back for my courage. Instead, he told me that he didn't want another 'needy' woman in his life. I was shocked. That wasn't at all what I was saying, but that's what he was hearing. From that experience, I think it's best to wait until the guy has a chance to know you better so that he doesn't jump to false conclusions about who you are and what you want from him."

Is there a definitive answer as to when is the "best" time to tell the man in your life about your breast cancer treatment? A good rule of thumb is: If you're in doubt, wait it out. But if you're genuinely confident and self-assured, why hesitate? Sooner is better, so go for it.

2. *Suppose you date a few times, tell him, and then get rejected?*

My personal reaction is "Good riddance." My professional response is that I'm very sorry you went through this painful experience. I'm also wondering if there were signals that you missed, or cues you avoided. Frequently, men give us valuable information about themselves without realizing it. And just as frequently, that information goes sailing right over our heads because we're oblivious to those cues. Learning how to be sensitive to relationship signals is a valuable asset for everyone and a particularly good skill for all breast cancer patients to acquire. In the meantime, I can guarantee that you won't go through this ordeal a second time if you use a technique that I call "taking his temperature."

Taking His Temperature

On the first or second date, casually mention that you just visited with a friend or relative who was recently treated for breast cancer. See what kind of reaction you get from him. How he responds will tell you a lot about the future of the relationship. If he changes the subject or clams up, you're in trouble. But if he asks intelligent questions and/or voluntarily tells you about a friend or relative who was successfully treated for breast cancer, you can be pretty certain that he's not cancerphobic and you've got a live one! This relationship has potential.

There is no question that "taking his temperature" is a manipulative strategy. But since it causes no harm or danger to anyone, and it protects you from investing your time and energy in a dead-end relationship, there is every reason to use it when you need to, or until you become more adept at reading cues and signals.

Some women take the guy's temperature on the first date and if the thermometer reads "normal," they tell him the rest of the story on the second date.

TAMMY casually mentioned on her first date with Ed that her best friend was going into the hospital the next day for a mastectomy and she (Tammy) was very concerned. Ed reassured her that one of the secretaries in his office had had a mastectomy ten years before and seemed to be doing fine. Tammy thought to herself, "so far so good." The following week, when they were at dinner, she told him that she had undergone a mastectomy and reconstruction several months before. Ed shrugged and said he kind of thought so, but was waiting for her to say something first. It was no big deal.

3. *When you have sex with him for the first time, do you have to let him see your breast?*

First-time sex for a couple is always awkward, even when breast cancer isn't an issue. Each of us is nervous. A man worries about the size of his penis and whether he will be able to perform. A woman worries about whether she looks sexy and how she can discreetly camouflage her stomach and thighs.

The anxiety doubles if the woman has also been treated for breast cancer. In addition to worrying about her stomach and thighs, she can now add breasts to the list.

Many women, married as well as single, prefer to wear a filmy nightgown or negligee the first time they make love. They may even continue to wear sexy lingerie every time thereafter. If the woman were not a breast cancer patient, no one would give this a second thought. Where is it written that, because you are a breast cancer patient, you have to bare your breasts in bed in order to prove to yourself, your partner, your doctors, and God knows who else that you have not rejected your femininity, sexuality, and womanhood?

The initial sexual encounter is difficult enough without the added worry of "How will he react to my breast?" If you have already told him about your surgery, you have taken the first and most important step. If you are uncomfortable revealing your breasts, I've got good news. There is no immediate need or reason to do it. It's perfectly sensible to wait until you are more comfortable in the relationship. For some of us it takes a few days, for others a few weeks, depending on the frequency of sex and your feelings about you, him, and the relationship.

You need to be reasonably comfortable with yourself in the nude before you can expect to be reasonably comfortable with *someone else seeing you* in the nude. Remember, if you were modest B.C., you're likely to be even more modest A.D. So if you're inclined to procrastinate, why not give yourself a practical plan to help you accomplish this goal? Here are two techniques that work:

The un-dress rehearsal

In the privacy of your own home, when you are alone, close the blinds, draw the drapes, and get naked! And while you are prancing about in your birthday suit, do some mundane chores like wash the dishes or vacuum the rug. Stay with it for a good half-hour and you will gradually begin to feel less self-conscious about your body. Give yourself as many un-dress rehearsals as you need.

Lights out

Wear a sexy negligee to bed and ask your partner to turn off the lights. Once it's dark, you will find it less intimidating for you and/or your partner to remove your negligee. You may choose to do this for days, weeks, or months. It's okay. Do it for as long as you need. With the passage of time and greater familiarity between the two of you, your inhibition will fade. Eventually, you will find yourself feeling comfortable in the nude with your partner, with the lights on or off.

I know there is an urgency to return to "normal" as soon as possible, but please go easy on yourself along the way. This is not a contest or a race. And if it were, then let's remember that it was the tortoise, not the hare, who won the race.

4. *If you had a lumpectomy/radiation procedure that is virtually undetectable, is it necessary to disclose this information to a prospective husband?*

I know there are plenty of women who lie to their husbands about their age, hair color, and nose job. So why should breast cancer be any different? Personally, I couldn't do it, it's not my style. But if *you* can and *you* want to, *I'll* never tell! However, I do think you need to keep in mind that what's sauce for the goose is sauce for the gander. Who knows what health secrets he's keeping from you!

Keeping your lumpectomy/radiation treatment a secret simply because you can get away with it is not such a great idea for other reasons as well. One of my patients, Mandy, was so obsessed with whether men could notice the difference in her radiated breast that she became sexually promiscuous.

> MANDY: "I realize now that I didn't really care about the men or the relationships. I just needed constant reassurance that my breasts were attractive and that men still found me desirable."

After a number of affairs, which, ironically, made her feel less secure about her sexual desirability, Mandy decided to get some professional help. As soon as she realized that attractiveness and desirability have to come from within, and that no one but you can give you this gift, she no longer found it necessary to jump into casual sexual relationships.

Sexual promiscuity isn't limited to women who have had lumpectomy/radiation treatment. Some of us with mastectomies (with or without reconstruction) become hypersexual, hoping to confirm our desirability. Needless to say, this is extremely self-destructive behavior, as well as dangerous.

5. *If he enjoys touching your reconstructed breast, do you confess that you have no feeling in it?*

Yes, but not while you're in the heat of passion, please. The time and place for this revelation is either before or after you make love, not during.

Because a reconstructed breast frequently looks and feels natural to your partner, he may assume that it looks and feels the same way to you. It can be confusing to a guy who hasn't been told the facts. He has no way of knowing that you have no sensation in that breast unless you tell him so.

Similarly, women with irradiated breasts find they are not as sensitive as they once were before treatment. How can your boyfriend possibly know this, when many of our own doctors aren't even aware?

This concern regarding breast sensitivity (or lack of it) is not limited to single women. Some of my married patients tell me that during lovemaking, their husbands forget and caress the reconstructed breast with great pleasure and excitement. Some women find this amusing, others think it's curious. I think it confirms something we've been told for years. Sexual excitation begins as a state of mind, not body.

If he enjoys your reconstructed breast, and you enjoy his enjoyment, why belabor the issue? If, however, you find it annoying or irritating, you need to discuss it openly or you will soon find yourself trumping up reasons to avoid sex.

Sexual fantasies

Somewhere along the way, you may find yourself having sexual fantasies or dreams about one or more of the doctors who are treating you. This can be pleasurable for some women but very alarming, even perturbing, for others, who may both fear and wish they will become sexually intimate with the doctor. Don't panic. You're not a pervert. This is a perfectly healthy and normal phenomenon. Two reasons it happens more frequently with our breast cancer doctors than it does with other physicians is: the relationship is extremely intense, and the breast is so closely linked to sexuality.

ANDREA was attractive, single, and in her early forties. Although she told me she was terrified of her diagnosis, the treatment, and her prognosis, all of our sessions were filled with talk of her sexual fantasies and attraction to her team of doctors, whom she called "The Magnificent Seven." She had the fear/wish that each would find out and either insist on consummating an affair with her—even though she felt that seven simultaneous affairs might be too promiscuous (a point well taken)—or worse, that all seven men would laugh at her attempts at seduction and not take her seriously. (Seven rejections in one fell swoop is a lot for anyone to handle, even if you're not battling breast cancer.)

The sexual fantasies started with the radiologist who discovered the lump on a mammogram, and soon included the surgeon and anesthesiologist. An oncologist came next, followed by a plastic surgeon and a radiation therapist. She accidentally met with the pathologist who had examined her breast tissue under the microscope and she fell for him as well. So Andrea loved seven doctors, all of whom were married, and none of whom had any idea of her secret longings. She could laugh about her fantasies in one moment and then, in the next, plummet into despair at the hopelessness of unrequited love for seven men. She wondered if they found her sexually desirable and searched for any small crumb of hope or shred of evidence that might confirm this.

Our sessions continued along in this manner, and I kept waiting for her to talk about the breast cancer. No way. Finally, I began to have serious concern for Andrea's seeming indifference to the reality of her diagnosis, treatment, and prognosis. Her preoccupation with sexual fantasies did not seem healthy. So I delicately broached the subject. Her response taught me more about human behavior than I learned in all of my doctoral training. Andrea looked at me and said, "Of course, I know that I'm using my sexual fantasies to avoid talking about my fears of breast cancer. What's so wrong about that? Don't you realize that my fantasies are the only pleasurable thing I have in my life right now? It's the only thing I have control over. The cancer and the doctors can take away my breast. But no one can take away my fantasies." I was stunned by the poignancy of her remarks and at how right she was. No matter what our diagnosis or prognosis may be, we all maintain control over our dreams and fantasies. Without them, life is meaningless. The only way Andrea could cope with the shock of her diagnosis and successfully get through the treatment (which she handled very well) was to construct a sexual fantasy world to retreat into when the fears and emotional strain were too much to handle. It never interfered with her going for treatment, and it didn't harm anyone. If anything, it helped her through a highly stressful and traumatic time in her life.

During the year that I saw her, Andrea became less fearful of her prognosis and more accepting of herself and the breast cancer. As she spoke more freely of her breast cancer fears, she began to lose romantic interest in her doctors. Ultimately, she found and connected with a "real live" boyfriend.

Is there a message here? You bet. There is no such thing as a bad or wrong sexual fantasy if it helps you through an ordeal and does not impede your treatment. Remember, the wish is not the deed. If it were, every one of us would be in prison!

Summary

The quality of the relationship between you and your partner is the key to sexual adjustment following breast cancer.

When the quality of the relationship is good, married women usually have an easier sexual adjustment than single women.

When the quality of the relationship is poor, married women usually have a more difficult sexual adjustment than single women.

Sexual adjustment after breast cancer is delicate and awkward, but doesn't have to be overwhelming. There are universal issues that are unavoidable and unnecessary issues that we can avoid.

You can improve your relationship or stop it from deteriorating further by learning how to communicate more effectively.

You and/or your partner's loss of interest in sex may be a result of depression, anger, and fear, rather than a reflection of your physical appearance.

Find time to be with your partner so that you have no intrusions. A weekend without kids or phones is perfect.

Don't stand on ceremony over who initiates sex first. What's more important is that you make love when you feel ready, not because you feel obligated to perform.

If your partner wants out of the relationship, he is most likely to leave at the time of diagnosis or after your treatment is over. He is least likely to leave while you're in treatment.

Single women have a special set of issues:

- To tell or not to tell on the first date.
- Coping with rejection from men.
- The initial sexual encounter and whether to reveal the mastectomy scar/reconstructed breast.
- Deciding whether to keep the lumpectomy/radiation treatment a secret from a lover.
- Deciding whether to disclose to a lover that there is little or no sensation in the treated breast.

Having sexual fantasies about our breast cancer doctors is normal and healthy. This phenomenon occurs for two reasons:
- The relationship is very intense.
- The breast is so closely linked to sexuality.

CHAPTER TEN

Coming to Terms With the Breast Cancer Experience: Residual Effects and Feelings

*C*oming to terms with the emotional impact of breast cancer is like sending in little David with his slingshot to conquer the giant Goliath. It looked impossible, even ludicrous, but by golly he did it! However, there is one major difference. Little David accomplished this feat in one shot. It will take us a tad longer.

The residual effects and feelings of our breast cancer odyssey fall into two basic categories: short term and long term. But on a more philosophical level, integrating our experience and coming to terms with it is an ongoing process that evolves over our lifetime. Whether we realize it or not, it's the residual effects and feelings that have a profound influence on our attitudes, interests, activities, and behavior.

The goal of this chapter is to prepare us to recognize, understand, and anticipate the residual effects and feelings we will encounter. That way, we won't be thrown for a loop, and, when possible, we will be able to resolve the issues ahead of time.

What are the short-term residual effects and feelings?

1. *Going cold turkey:* This is a universal, unavoidable condition that all chemotherapy/radiation patients experience. It's a funny thing, no matter how much we look forward to the last day of treatment, when it ends, it is such an abrupt change in our life and shock to our system that we suffer withdrawal symptoms. One of my patients summed it up this way:

> "I got used to the set routine and the schedule. I knew what to expect and how I would feel. The day after the treatment ended, instead of feeling elated, I felt anxious because now I had this big empty void in my life and I didn't know how to fill it. I actually broke out in a cold sweat."

Another stated:

> "Radiation therapy doesn't taper off slowly. It's all or nothing. You're either in it or you're not. And when mine ended, I really missed it. Not so much the treatment, but the *idea* of the treatment. I was afraid that without ongoing radiation, the cancer would recur."

And last but not least:

"Sure, the chemo made me sick, but I felt like I was actively doing something to control the disease. Now that the treatment is over, I've got nothing to take its place. It seems like I'm waiting for the other shoe to drop. I don't like the feeling."

Feeling empty and lost without treatment and fearing a recurrence are usually accompanied by the belief that unless we see the doctor frequently, we won't survive very well on our own.

2. *The Lone Soldier Syndrome:* When the dust settles and the smoke clears, it becomes apparent that no doctors or technicians are hovering around us anymore. We are left to our own devices. Except for periodic checkups, there is only one soldier left on the battlefield—you! It feels like an impossible and heavy burden!

"I was like a baby bird that got kicked out of the nest before anyone knew if it could fly."

"I felt so incompetent. I didn't know how to effectively monitor my recovery and health between checkups. What was I supposed to be looking for? And how would I know if I found it?"

"I wasn't ready to go out there alone. I felt abandoned and rejected by my doctors. On one level I knew this was ridiculous, but on another level I wasn't so sure."

It's hard to say which is more anxiety-provoking: abruptly ending the treatment or giving up the army of medical people who monitor our progress.

Both the Lone Soldier Syndrome and Going Cold Turkey respond very favorably to group therapy. There we will find other lone soldiers who have gone cold turkey and, like ourselves, are looking for reassurance, camaraderie, safety, and a place to ask questions and vent feelings.

Knowing what to expect when our chemotherapy/radiation or surgery is over can eliminate some of the discomfort when the event actually takes place. And it gives us the advance opportunity to find a breast cancer support group, if we haven't already located one.

What if you can't find a support group in your town? I have two suggestions: a) Talk to some of the local doctors and ask if they will help you contact other women with the same needs; b) Go to the public relations department of your community hospital and ask if they will put together a breast cancer group as a public service. Frequently, if the doctors are interested, the hospital will sponsor the group and find an appropriate leader.

3. *The Privileged Character Syndrome.* During treatment, our family and friends fussed over us and made us feel like V.I.P.s. Now that the treatment is over and we're able to function effectively, we are no longer "Queen for a Day." We're expected to pass on the crown and mantle to someone else (or at the very least, take the damn thing off and put it in the closet). Ah, but life isn't that simple. Once you've tasted privilege, you hate to part with it. Even Cinderella tarried a bit at the ball before returning to her life as a scullery maid.

Now it's very unlikely that your daily life is that of a scullery maid. But sometimes it feels that way. And the more it does, the more reluctant we are to give up the royal treatment.

Some of the symptoms of the Privileged Character Syndrome include:

1. *Making excessive demands on family and friends.*

"What do you mean, you can't stay on the phone to chat?"

(Psychological interpretation: I'm lonely and need some company, but I'm too ashamed to tell you.)

"Why won't you leave work a little early to pick me up at the hairdresser?"

(Psychological interpretation: This is a test to see how much you love me. If you *really* love me, you will put your needs aside and concentrate on my needs. And even if you do, I will continue to test you until you finally fail.)

2. *Insisting on having your own way, even in trivial matters.*

"If we don't go first class, I simply won't go."

(Psychological interpretation: I don't feel very good or confident about who I am. This is how I disguise it and get people to think I'm special.)

"Twelve o'clock is too early for lunch. I can't eat before twelve fifteen."

(Psychological interpretation: If I can't control the breast cancer, I'm going to control the relationship with you.)

Before we alienate our loved ones with unreasonable demands, why not find ways to gratify these needs in a more positive way? For example, make new friends who share similar concerns, explore new projects, join interesting organizations or groups. Line up some pleasurable activities before your treatment ends, so that you will have something enjoyable to look forward to. That way, you won't feel like you're giving up all of the good to return to all of the bad. And if your life really is all that bad (or at least feels that way to you), now is the time to get some professional help.

What are the long-term residual effects and feelings?

1. *We have a nose for news that never ends.*
If it pertains to breast cancer, just ask us. We'll quote

you which newspaper, edition, page number, and writer. It's ironic that when we think we've got a handle on every anxiety-provoking issue and situation that could possibly occur, somebody throws us a curve ball. Specifically, who wasn't unnerved, if not downright panicked, when we read that as few as three alcoholic beverages a week increase the risk for breast cancer. Each of us mentally skimmed the pages of our past, feverishly counting the number of glasses of wine we quaffed last night, last week, last month, last year, and the last decade. And we wondered if, some-how, that one extra Martini, Margarita, or Long Island Iced Tea might have been the culprit, the decisive factor in our developing breast cancer.

No sooner did we come to terms with how much we did or didn't drink in the past, and how much we will or won't drink in the future, when we were hit with another new wrinkle that we didn't anticipate: Breast enlargement (sili-cone implants) may mask early detection of breast cancer. (Mammograms cannot see behind the implants, where an early cancer may be growing.) That piece of unpleasant news caused alarm in every woman with breast implants who was later treated for breast cancer.

Because breast cancer is such a hot topic, there is hardly a week that goes by without some new and startling piece of information. If we read every word of it, we will have no time left for the fun things in life. If we believe every word of it, we will make ourselves crazy.

For example, LYNNE was one month postmastectomy when she read an article on how fat in the diet increases breast cancer risk. On the verge of tears, she told her weekly support group, "I love ice cream but I'm never going to eat it again. Last night, I ate a scoop of my favorite flavor, looked at my children, and cried. I realized I was jeopardizing my life and sacrificing my children for the sake of an ice cream cone. How could I make ice cream more important than living to see my babies grow up?"

This is exactly the kind of thinking that takes all the joy

out of life and makes us feel guilty for every small pleasure. After some group discussion, Lynne was able to put the concept of low-fat diet into proper perspective and was less critical of herself. She allowed as how an occasional ice cream treat would not shorten her life.

Granted, a low-fat diet is preferable to high fat, but that doesn't mean that you never again eat ice cream, cheese, or other dairy products. It means that you reduce your fat intake to a level that satisfies your craving without "pigging out." If you eat conservatively and in moderation, you can enjoy *all foods* without feeling guilty.

The same for alcohol. If you're on the wagon, or want to go on it, please don't let me stop you. But if you enjoy a glass of wine with dinner, now is the time to give yourself permission to relax, enjoy your meal, and not feel like a convicted felon who's headed for the electric chair.

2. *What was yesterday's truth is today's trash.*

Theoretically, it is reassuring to know there is so much interest and scientific research going on in the breast cancer field. But on a practical level, it's very traumatic to be informed, on what amounts to a weekly basis, that so many of the things that used to be good and safe are now bad or suspect for breast cancer. In other words, the frequency with which yesterday's truth is turning into today's trash is rather disconcerting. Instead of reducing our anxiety and causing us to rejoice that the prevention and cure for breast cancer are just around the corner, it often has the opposite effect. It leaves us feeling discouraged, cynical, angry, and wary of the medical profession.

YVETTE: "When I was a teenager I had acne on my face and chest that left scars. I always felt self-conscious, and finally, after I was married, I decided to do something about it. I had radiation treatment that my doctor assured me was safe. Twenty-five years later they found out that the treatment is probably what contributed to, if not caused, my breast cancer.

I am furious with myself for being so vain that I elected unnecessary cosmetic treatment, equally furious with that doctor for telling me that it was safe when it turned out later that it wasn't, depressed that I got breast cancer, and guilty for putting my family through the past six months of chemotherapy."

It was easy for me to see Yvette's point of view and understand her anger. During the course of her psychotherapy, she resolved many of her negative feelings and came to terms with the rage toward herself, the situation, and the medical profession. She grew to realize that each of us does the best we can, based on what we believe is the truth. Our doctors do the same. To spend the rest of our lives torturing ourselves for having made what seemed to be a wise and healthy choice at the time is a waste of energy. Nobody can second-guess life and its vicissitudes. Carry that to its logical conclusion and none of us would ever make a decision about anything again (including whether to get out of bed in the morning) for fear of the possible negative consequences.

As breast cancer patients, this is a particularly significant point to keep in mind. Why? Because as science comes up with new findings, the facts and the "truth" change. These changes may very well impact the quality and quantity of our lives . . . for better or worse. Either way, it's important to remember that our doctors are doing the best they can with the available "truth." Win, lose, or draw, all that any of us can do is give it our best shot.

3. *Statistics are sadistic.*

While we're on the subject of second-guessing the future, I'm reminded of another issue that petrifies most of us. Survival statistics. I wish for the mental health of every breast cancer patient that the statistical tables of survival probability were wiped off the face of the earth. They do nothing but raise our anxiety level and cause unnecessary emotional turmoil, and they are meaningless when applied to any one individual.

I know there is enormous temptation to find out what the long-term survival probability is for your type of breast cancer. But it's like Pandora's Box—if you insist on lifting the lid, you'll only give yourself a lot of aggravation and no peace of mind.

For argument's sake, let's say you go ahead anyway and find out your probabilities. Hypothetically, you discover that your chances for survival are eighty percent. Does it say whether you're in the eighty percent group that will survive, or the twenty percent group that won't? No. So what have you found out? Not much. But just enough to give you a whole bunch of meaningless numbers and percentages to bat around in your head until you drive yourself to distraction. Can you psychologically afford to take on another avoidable problem in your life? Then don't.

One last thought on the subject: Regardless of the size and type of the tumor, or the nature of the treatment you receive, you have a survival probability of either one hundred percent or zero. Think about that. You either live or you die. There ain't nothing in between. So if you insist on playing the odds, why not bet on yourself to win?

4. *Today it's unique, tomorrow antique.*

Improvements and innovations in treatment techniques may one day make our treatment choice old hat. In other words, what is state-of-the-art today, tomorrow could be passé. If and when this happens to us, it's perfectly normal to feel sad and envious, and wish that we had been able to avail ourselves of the newer treatment.

For instance, there are some women who would have preferred lumpectomy-radiation had it been available at the time of their diagnoses. Although they are grateful to

be alive, and have comfortably accepted their mastectomies, there is still the wish that the timing had been
different. Similarly, those of us who underwent lumpec-
tomy/radiation in the early years may not be thrilled with
the cosmetic results, and consequently we envy those who
followed in our footsteps and whose cosmetic results are
beautiful.

5. *Getting in gear for your once-a-year.*

Working up to the yearly mammogram and routine
followup visit is a major production. We're talking jumbo
jitters. Galloping insomnia. Loss of appetite or stuffing
your face (whichever you do best). It's not unusual to make
the appointment months in advance so that we can "prepare" for the event (not unlike a boxer going into training). It's also not unusual to cancel on the day of the
appointment because we haven't "prepared" enough
(we're too scared to show up).

Incidentally, for the first year or two following treatment, you will be seen more frequently than once a year.
What this means is you have more opportunities to either
psych out or *psych up*. The former you know how to do very
well without my assistance. So here are some ways to *psych
up* for the visit:

• Use your support group or individual therapy to
vent your anxiety. In return, the group members will
bolster your confidence and spirit.

• Invest in some relaxation tapes and play them
two to three times a day. Learning how to do self-
hypnosis and guided imagery can help reduce anxiety and fear.

• Buy yourself a small gift or plan some joyful event
following your appointment, as a reward for your

courage. (Why do you think pediatricians hand out lollipops?)

6. *The itch and the twitch are really a bitch.*

Welcome to the world of hypochondria! We've been expecting you. The day your treatment ends is the day you become a vigilante committee of one on the prowl for any sniffle, sneeze, itch, or twitch that could possibly signal "something." "Something" invariably turns out to be your period or a touch of the flu.

For the first couple of years, you're apt to run to the doctor as soon as a symptom of any kind surfaces. After a while, you start feeling like a damn fool running from one specialist to the next, so you decide to lighten up. This is a great idea, because it immediately frees you to spend your time and money on fun activities. Go for it!

7. *It's better not to give or receive.*

Once we are treated for breast cancer, what is the genetic likelihood of passing it on to future generations?

- We worry that if we decide to have children, we may inadvertently give the "bad seed" to our daughters.

- We fear that if we already have daughters, they have already received the "bad seed" from us.

- If our daughters do develop breast cancer, we feel guilty.

- If we are the daughter who received the "bad seed" from our mother, we feel betrayed, and then guilty for feeling that way about Mom.

What can we do to reduce the stress and tension?
If you are the mother, encourage your daughter to

meet with a breast cancer specialist who will decide which tests, if any, are indicated at this time. In addition, the specialist will discuss breast health with her, answer questions, dispel myths, and raise her consciousness without scaring her.

If you are the daughter, encourage your mother to meet with you, and together go to a psychotherapist to discuss and resolve the feelings of betrayal and guilt that both of you feel toward each other. If your mother is deceased, or refuses to join you in therapy, you can still work on these issues and resolve them for yourself.

Not every long-term residual effect and feeling is a problem. Here are some of the benefits and advantages:

8. *You don't need a watch to tell time.*

Breast cancer gives us a greater awareness of time and our own mortality. We are able to stop putting off for tomorrow what is pleasurable today. We look forward to the future, but we live in the present. Tomorrow is good, the here and now is better . . . especially when you're doing what you like with people you love.

> "We were going to wait for summer to visit our grandchildren. But we decided to send for them over Easter vacation. We can still go there in July, too."

> "I've been wanting to learn how to scuba dive since I was a kid, but my father thought it was too dangerous. Last week, my boyfriend and I signed up for a trip to Tahiti where they're going to teach us."

9. *You can sort out the sense from the nonsense.*

Peering into the jaws of death gives us a fresh perspective on life. We acquire a new sensibility about ourselves and what we need. Suddenly, we are focused. It's clear what's important and what's trivial. We put our priorities in order without feeling remorse or the need to explain. We know it's okay to keep the best and toss the rest.

"I like my job a lot, but I like my family more. I'm not going to work weekends again."

"I've always wanted to live at the beach overlooking the water, but the rent is so expensive. Today I decided I'm worth it."

10. *You know when to hold 'em, and when to fold 'em.*
I'm talking about relationships. We find the necessary courage to finally end relationships that don't work and replace them with new ones that do.

"I was in a bad marriage for years. Both of us were miserable and didn't have the guts to do anything about it. I decided I could not spend the rest of my life—be it five years or fifty—that unhappy. I'm now divorced, and dating a man I love and who loves me. Had I not been treated for breast cancer, I doubt that I would have had the strength to put an end to a marriage that died years ago, and go out and find someone else."

11. *You know how to survive in a storm.*
Our ship got caught in the eye of the hurricane and made us fear for our lives. It left us a bit battered and scarred, but miraculously we emerged in one piece and still afloat. No, we didn't sail through the diagnosis and treatment, but we did hang in there! And let's face it, there were days when we had serious doubts. What did we gain from weathering the storm? A feeling of inner strength, power, and the knowledge that we are *SURVIVORS!* Once we have gained this feeling, it is ours forever. We will be able to use it again, whenever we want or need it.

Yes, we have Damocles' sword hanging over our heads. But you know what? So does everyone. Every human being is going to die and no one knows exactly when, where, or how. As breast cancer survivors, we have been grazed by the sword. It left us with physical and psychological wounds. We have two choices. We can do what is necessary to heal the wounds. Or we can let the injuries fester until they make the rest of our life painful and uncomfortable. We can either turn our back on life and have it end before we're ready, or make the most of life by seizing each day and making it count for something. The choice is ours.

It is unrealistic to think we will not experience both negative as well as positive residual effects. We all do. But whether we spend more time and energy dwelling on the negative instead of the positive depends on our feelings of self-worth and our willingness to take a lemon and make lemonade. Breast cancer is one of life's lemons. Don't let it sour the rest of your life. Become psychologically aware of your feelings and the various ways breast cancer has impacted your life. Then go talk it through with a licensed psychotherapist or in a support group. Not only will it help you cope more effectively, but it's also my professional trade secret for making lemonade!

I hope this book will help you in healing the emotional wounds that leave *invisible scars.*

Appendix A

Suggested Reading List

Belsky, Marvin S., M.D., and Leonard Gross. *How to Choose and Use Your Doctor*. New York: Arbor House, 1979. Some pointers on getting good medical care.

Berger, Karen, and John Bostich III, M.D. *A Woman's Decision: Breast Care, Treatment and Reconstruction*. St. Louis, Mo.: C.V. Mosby, 1984. An objective overview of treatments for breast cancer, with a strong focus on reconstruction and several personal stories.

Brody, Jane. *Jane Brody's Nutrition Book*. New York: Norton, 1981. Paperback edition, Bantam, 1982. A comprehensive, thorough guide to nutrition and weight control.

Bruning, Nancy. *Coping with Chemotherapy: How to Take Care of Yourself While Chemotherapy Takes Care of the Cancer*. New York: Doubleday, 1985. Paperback edition, Ballantine, 1986. Everything you want to know about chemotherapy by a breast cancer patient who experienced the treatment firsthand.

Budoff, Penny Wise, M.D. *No More Hot Flashes and Other Good News*. New York: G.P. Putnam's Sons, 1983. Revised paperback edition, Warner, 1984. Required reading for every woman over thirty-five who wants to understand what's happening to her body as well as how and why; excellent chapter on breast cancer treatment options.

Butler, Robert, and Myrna Lewis. *Love and Sex After Forty*.

New York: Harper and Row, 1986. A revised edition of their earlier title, *Love and Sex After Sixty* (1976), this book, like the earlier one, discusses many aspects of sexuality and addresses issues relevant to cancer patients.

Carrera, Michael. *Sex: The Facts, the Acts, and Your Feelings.* New York: Crown, 1981. Good suggestions for those whose sexual performance has been altered by surgery, as well as a full discussion of all aspects of sex and sexuality.

Fiore, Neil A. *The Road Back to Health: Coping with the Emotional Side of Cancer.* New York: Bantam, 1984. The author, a former cancer patient, focuses on how to cope with cancer.

Harrington, Gerri. *The Health Insurance Fact and Answer Book.* New York: Harper and Row, 1985. An excellent guide to group, individual, disability, and indemnity policies for anyone, including those who have Medicare.

Kelly, Sean F., Ph.D., and Reid J. Kelly, A.C.S.W. *Hypnosis: Understanding How It Can Work for You.* Reading, Mass.: Addison-Wesley, 1985. An introduction for professionals and the general public on the clinical applications of hypnosis. The section on hypnosis and medicine for the control of pain is very useful.

Kushner, Rose. *Alternatives: New Developments in the War on Breast Cancer.* Cambridge, Mass.: Kensington Press, 1984. Formerly published as *Why Me?*, it has been updated from her 1976 and 1982 books in which this medical journalist wrote about her experiences with her own mastectomy and gave important medical information. This new book describes her most recent research in the treatment of recurring breast cancer. The most definitive book on the subject for lay people; somewhat technical.

Margie, Joyce Daly, M.S., and Abby S. Block, M.S., R.D. *Nutrition and the Cancer Patient.* Radnor, Pa.: Chilton,

1983. Background information, specific problems, practical solutions, and recipes are included.

Nierenberg, Judith, R.N., and Florence Janovic. *The Hospital Experience*. New York: Berkley, 1985. An expanded and updated version of their 1978 book, this is a complete guide to understanding and participating in your own care; an essential book for every home library.

Pepper, Curtis Bill. *We the Victors: Inspiring Stories of People Who Conquered Cancer and How They Did It*. New York: Doubleday, 1984. An in-depth report on people who survived cancer; what they believe to have been crucial to their recovery and how the disease has changed their lives.

Siegel, Bernie S., M.D. *Love, Medicine and Miracles: Lessons Learned About Self-Healing from a Surgeon's Experience with Exceptional Patients*. New York: Harper and Row, 1986. Explores the relationship between attitude and disease, and mind-body interaction.

Siegel, Mary-Ellen. *The Cancer Patient's Handbook*. New York: Walker and Company, 1986. A ready-reference guide to the range of medical and emotional concerns facing cancer patients, their families, and friends, written in an easy-to-understand style.

Simonton, O. Carl, M.D., Stephanie Matthews-Simonton, and James L. Creighton. *Getting Well Again*. New York: Bantam, 1980. Many patients find this book very helpful in acquiring positive attitudes, relaxation and pain management, while others claim that it evokes guilt and self-blame.

Snyder, Marilyn. *An Informed Decision: Understanding Breast Reconstruction*. New York: Evans, 1984. The author, a writer and actress, explains breast reconstruction.

Sontag, Susan. *Illness as Metaphor*. New York: Farrar, Straus & Giroux, 1977. Paperback edition, Vintage Books, 1979. A perceptive book that cuts through the cultural interpretations of serious illness and analyzes social attitudes toward major illnesses, including cancer.

Spletter, Mary. *A Woman's Choice*. Boston: Beacon Press, 1982. Good general information on breast cancer treatment with detailed information on breast reconstruction; combines her own experience with stories of other women.

Tatelbaum, Judy. *The Courage to Grieve*. New York: Lippencott & Crowell, 1980. A guide to creative living, recovery, and growth through grief.

Viorst, Judith. *Necessary Losses*. New York: Simon & Schuster, 1986. Insights and interpretations of loss and subsequent gains that draw on psychoanalytic theories of child development and the writings of poets and philosophers.

The following excellent books and a list of other publications are available free from:

> Office of Cancer Communications
> National Cancer Institute
> Building 31, Room 10A18
> Bethesda, MD 20205

The Breast Cancer Digest. Written primarily for health-care providers, this frank and comprehensive book discusses diagnosis, treatment, and recovery; the survival statistics may be off-putting to the newly diagnosed/treated.

Chemotherapy and You. An easy-to-read guide to self-help during treatment.

Breast Cancer Patient Education Series. A series of well-written booklets that discuss treatment options: mastectomy, radiation therapy, and adjuvant chemotherapy.

The NCI will also send you a list of other breast cancer publications and booklets; all of them are frequently updated, and occasionally new ones are published.

Appendix B

Suggested Audiotapes

Boornstein, Diana Longstreet; Golde, Marcia; Silk, Ellen. *A Matter of Choice: Treatment Options for Breast Cancer.* Distributed by Healthcomm, 1985. P.O. Box 5475, Sherman Oaks, CA 91403. A reassuring and easy-to-use two-part audio cassette program designed for home use to inform patients about treatment options for breast cancer.

For free catalogs that list tape recordings of relaxation and guided imagery, write to the following three companies:

> Psychology Today Tapes
> Box 059061
> Brooklyn, NY 11205-9061

Among the tapes available from Psych Today are: "Learning to Control Pain" (which focuses on guided imagery); "What Is Hypnosis, and What Can It Do for Me?"; "Two Exercises in Hypnosis"; "Progressive Relaxation"; and "Deep Relaxation and Meditation: An Instructional Cassette."

> Guilford Publications, Inc.
> 200 Park Avenue South
> New York, NY 10003

The audiotapes available from Guilford include: "Passive Muscle Relaxation"; "Personal Enrichment Through Imagery"; "Principles and Practice of Progressive Relaxation: A Teaching Primer"; "Quieting Reflex Training for Adults"; "Relaxation Techniques"; "Relaxation Training Program"; and "Self-Transformation Through the New Hypnosis."

Carle Medical Communications
510 West Main Street
Urbana, IL 61801

An excellent videotape and audiotape, both entitled "Controlling the Behavioral Side Effects of Chemotherapy" (including exercises in passive relaxation) are available.

Appendix C

Organizations of Interest

The National Alliance of Breast Cancer Organizations (NABCO) serves as a central information bank for a variety of breast cancer interest groups and organizations that offer emotional support, current research, legislative reform, and general information. Individual as well as group memberships are welcomed.

> The National Alliance of Breast Cancer
> Organizations
> Second Floor
> 1180 Avenue of the Americas
> New York, NY 10036
> 212-719-0154

The National Cancer Institute conducts its own breast cancer research. Especially useful and valuable to breast cancer patients and their families is NCI's information and referral service. This service is called the Cancer Information Service (CIS) of the National Cancer Institute. The toll-free phone numbers to reach them are:

In the continental United States (except the Washington, D.C., area): 1-800-4-CANCER.

In Hawaii: 808-524-1234 (local in Oahu; from neighboring islands, call collect)

In Washington, D.C., (and suburbs in Maryland and Virginia): 202-636-5700.

In Alaska: 1-800-638-6070.

When you call the CIS number, you are connected with the regional office serving your area. They can give you accurate, personalized answers to your breast cancer questions, and can tell you about various community agencies and services available.

The American Cancer Society, in addition to funding research, sponsors several patient-support programs for breast cancer patients, such as Reach To Recovery. Look in your local telephone directory for the nearest ACS division or unit. They can give you information about locally available services and provide you with various written materials. If you are unable to find the local division, contact the national office:

American Cancer Society
National Headquarters
90 Park Avenue
New York, NY 10016
212-599-8200

Index